Healing and Treatment of Diseases Through Water

Indian Medical Science Series No. 19

Healing and Treatment of Diseases Through Water

Sebastian Kneipp

Sri Satguru Publications
A Division of
Indian Books Centre
Delhi - India

Published by
Sri Satguru Publications,
Indological and Oriental Publishers
A Division of
Indian Books Centre
40/5, Shakti Nagar,
Delhi-110007
India

Email: ibcindia@vsnl.com
Website: http://www.indianbookscentre.com

Second Revised Edition; Delhi 1996
Reprinted ; 2007

ISBN 81-7030-494-6

Printed at Chawla Offset Printers, Delhi 110 052

CONTENTS.

TRANSLATOR'S PREFACE.

THE little German volume, of which this is a translation, is the record of a system of water-cure practised for over sixteen years by Sebastian Kneipp, the parish priest of Wörishofen in Bavaria, with such remarkable success that it has attracted notice all over Europe, and drawn thither invalids from the remotest corners of the Continent as well as from England. In this work Pfarrer Kneipp relates how gradually he reduced his own experiences with cold water to a settled system—the one by means of which he has cured and is daily curing thousands of patients. Not all at once did his knowledge come; for long he groped about in the dark, and as he himself confesses, had to remodel his system completely, no less than three times. For thirty years he made of water his study, verifying each separate prescription on his own person over and over again, before he presumed to set himself up as a healer of men; and his actual system has now been proved and vindicated by full fifteen years' successful practice.

At first he only aspired to curing his own parishioners, but his fame grew apace, bringing him from far and wide patients of every description and rank of life, afflicted with every possible manner of disease. His name has become a household word throughout Germany and Austria: his photograph is displayed in every shop-window; and "Pfarrer Kneipp" bread, coffee, and linen are everywhere advertised by wide-awake speculators who seek to make capital out of his popularity.

The writer's maxims and prescriptions are expressed with an almost childish simplicity, not to call it rusticity, of language, which is, however, the book's greatest charm. You cannot help feeling, as you read it, that this man owes nothing to the teachings of science, but everything to an inborn gift, so strongly developed as almost to deserve the name of inspiration. No technical terms, no learnedly incomprehensible medicinal phrases, are here employed to illustrate his meaning; but a simple child of nature himself, he borrows his similes from "the common growth of mother earth" around him.

The translator has sought as much as possible to preserve the simple and homely style of the original work, and though some of the terms do not answer strictly to their restricted meanings in English medical nomenclature, they will not the less convey their import with sufficient clearness to readers in general. The author does not write in medical phraseology; his object is to give a plain account of his treatment in popular language; and the translator has endeavoured to preserve as much as possible this feature in the English translation.

As the original German work contains numerous superfluous repetitions, occasional curtailments have been considered necessary in order to adapt the book to the exigencies of the British public. This has chiefly taken place when the author, having described several parallel instances of cure from the identical complaint, the translator has selected for exemplification the case or cases which seemed most deserving of notice.

Having the advantage of being personally acquainted with the author of this quaint volume, and having derived much benefit from his treatment, some personal impressions of himself and his establishment may not be inappropriate. It is now several years ago since a friend accidentally mentioned to me that, somewhere in Bavaria, there lived an old country priest who had cured many people by a most simple mode of treatment, in which cold water was chiefly used, applied in a quite original manner—very different from the mode adopted by Priessnitz and his successors. Two or three years passed by, without my further hearing of him. Meanwhile I had been a dreadful sufferer from that bane of the present century—nerves; and though I had consulted doctors innumerable, the result had always been that I was patched up for a time; and it was only latterly, at a moment when I was particularly depressed by an aggravated return of my old symptoms, that Pfarrer Kneipp's name was again brought before me. By this time it was evident either that the doctors had failed to discover the real evil, or that their remedies, strong as they were, could not help me. I first sent an account of my symptoms, and asked whether my case was one likely to be benefited by his treatment. I received no answer. This rather discouraged me, and I was nearly abandoning my newly formed project, when I heard that the Pfarrer had been obliged to give up even opening letters on account of the immense numbers which reached him. My curiosity was now powerfully roused, and I thought it worth while to go out of my way to see for myself. Accordingly, one hot July forenoon, after an hour and a half's journey from Munich, I found myself at Buchloe, one of the stations for Worishofen, and I started off for the village in the lumbering old carriage which awaited me.

As I had been warned that it was very difficult to procure accommodation, I had prudently secured a room beforehand through the kindness of some friends who had been there. It was rather startling, however, to find two students already in possession, and I had yet to learn what a precious thing a room was in this little village of Wörishofen, where hundreds congregated, putting up cheerfully with every discomfort. In the meantime here I was in the street with my boxes, and as I watched the carriage disappearing in the distance, I could not help wishing I had followed my doctor's advice, and that I was now installed in the Baierischer Hof at Lindau, with the beautiful Lake of Constance before me.

Wörishofen, whose inhabitants number about 1400, and its houses 180, is neither beautiful nor picturesque: there are fine pine-woods with undergrowth of beech within twenty minutes' walk of the place; but otherwise the country round is flat and uninteresting, and the village itself exceedingly commonplace, exactly resembling a dozen other Bavarian villages I had previously seen. Yet no stranger can put foot in the village street without at once being aware that this place is not as other places, being animated throughout by some pervading spirit, which finds expression in every detail of indoor and outdoor life. The whole village appears to be decked out with a profusion of snowy pennons, which on a windy day flutter in the air as though a universal truce had been proclaimed by mankind; on the paling of each little garden that faces the street may be seen dripping sheets and towels hung there to dry; wet linen shirts and inexpressibles, suspended on ropes, dance gaily in the breeze like rows of cheerful spectres; and each open window-casement is stuck full to overflowing with bedding in every stage of moisture. Numerous town-clad people are sauntering about the roads, mostly without collar or necktie, and often without their boots, which they carry in the hand in as natural and matter-of-fact a manner as we are wont to carry our parasols and walking-sticks. Wörishofen is the feet's paradise, according to Pfarrer Kneipp, who says: "How must the poor feet rejoice to come out at last from their cages and feel the rays of the warm sunshine! Fain would they never go back to their dark prisons!"

Invalid priests and monks make up a large proportion of the guests at Wörishofen. Almost every variety of religious attire may be seen here, from the purple robe of the church dignitary to the coarse brown dress of the mendicant friar. They are afflicted with every manner of disease, and speak in every kind of strange tongue.

When I had taken stock of these immediate surroundings, my next step was naturally to seek an interview with the man on whose account I had come so far. Despite all I had heard about the press of visitors, I was not prepared to find this so difficult a matter as it proved to be; and when I saw the numbers of people all waiting patiently around his house, I began for the first time to realise that here was something quite out of the common.

At last he made his appearance, a white-haired old man of imposing figure, and with a powerful face, to which specially dark bushy eyebrows gave peculiar character. Despite the excessive simplicity of his attire, there was something positively majestic about him. I wish I could put him before my readers as he stands vividly before my mind's eye. I am almost at a loss to explain or account for the deep impression which he made upon me—and upon others as well, as I have frequently heard—but I think the secret of his power lies in the eyes, looking out at one as they do from the shadow of those prominent brows: above all, one is struck by the upward look they sometimes have. Instead of fixing his eyes straight on the patient as he speaks, they are slightly upraised, as though he beheld something unseen by us, and were drawing from above the inspiration which would dictate his answer. Now and again he will turn his gaze full on the patient in a manner calculated to render nervous any one who does not rejoice in a quiet conscience—for at such times his eye looks as though it could penetrate the inmost workings of the soul.

Quite remarkable, too, is the unerring rapidity with which he forms his conclusions. He asks few questions, and refuses to listen to any long-winded account of symptoms; but gives his instructions with a briefness and rapidity quite bewildering to the uninitiated. In some cases this seemed so striking that I felt that a total stranger stepping in, and being a witness of one of these semi-public consultations, would say, here must be a great charlatan or a great genius. One must, however, judge by results; and turn where you may, you hear of the marvellous cures effected by him. What seemed to me so marvellous and admirable was the perfect and fearless confidence which inspired every word he said, and at the same time the utter absence of all self-consciousness, as if he considered this wonderful power which lay in him to be something independent of himself,—something of which he was merely the keeper and dispenser.

He specially prides himself on the simplicity of his cure, which renders it accessible to the poorest—and here lies his true vocation, helping the poor. While he is kind to every one, it is easy to see that his whole heart goes out to meet those who are in want.

After a much varied experience of visits to celebrated doctors, and endless weary hours misspent in stereotyped waiting-rooms, turning over the pages of the inevitable illustrated newspapers and albums, *de rigueur* at such places, the surroundings here were refreshingly unconventional. The *Pfarrhof*[1] stands in the centre of the village, within a courtyard, whose gate leading on to the road is locked, as protection against the press of visitors, who were thus supposed to ring for admittance: few people, however, took the trouble to do so, having quickly discovered that it was far simpler to go round through the churchyard and garden, whence one could enter the house unchallenged. A large passage or lobby runs through the *Pfarrhof* from end to end. Here the patients

[1] Parsonage or rectory.

used to assemble, even consultations often being held here with Arcadian simplicity and publicity—most of the simple-minded country people seeming to experience no embarrassment in relating their symptoms and receiving directions before the whole assembly of mixed sexes.

Though, as a rule, I preferred to take advantage of the privilege accorded me of going up to the Pfarrer's private sitting-room for my consultations, yet I liked to assist occasionally at these public assemblies, which were often very entertaining. One day, for instance, when describing to a female patient the appearance of a certain flower to be used as remedy, provoked at her ignorance on the subject, he exclaimed: "You women have got your heads covered up with gaudy flowers; but when it is a question of recognising a useful one, you know nothing about it!" As this happened to be in summer, when straw hats, trimmed profusely with flowers, were growing rank on every head, there was of course a titter of amusement from the male portion of the audience.

Another time it was a showy bracelet composed of gold links which challenged his animosity. "Have you a dog?" he suddenly apostrophised the lady, whose misfortune it was to be thus decorated. Then receiving no answer but a bewildered stare, he proceeded, "If you have no dog, then why carry a chain about with you?—take it off at once."

The window-sills of this lobby were heaped with huge bundles of herbs, which shed a faint aromatic perfume throughout the atmosphere, while bottles containing liquid decoctions of the same, stood about promiscuously; and though I never saw a label or ticket upon either bundle or bottle, yet the Pfarrer did not seem to find the slightest difficulty in identifying his remedies. Likewise his *soutane* pockets seemed endless in their resources, apparently harbouring the contents of a whole apothecary's shop; for, frequently consulted by patients in the village street or the road, he invariably happened to have about his person the precise remedy demanded by their condition.

Strangers coming here were apt at first to be somewhat startled at the unconventionality of Pfarrer Kneipp's proceedings; as was the case with a young English friend of mine with whom I happened to be walking on the first evening of her arrival at Wörishofen. As we passed through the main street of the village, we chanced to meet the Pfarrer walking with another gentleman. Without checking his pace, and almost without glancing in our direction, he dived his hand into the pocket of his *soutane* and produced a small bottle, which he thrust into my hand as he passed, merely muttering as he did so, "Fifty drops in eight spoonfuls of water twice daily," and then walked on, resuming the conversation which had scarcely been interrupted by his action.

My friend was evidently much bewildered, till I explained that this must probably refer to a question I had put to the good Pfarrer at the very early hour of 6 A.M.; and considering the circumstance that he must have seen some hundred and fifty patients in the interval, and that I never saw him make a note or memorandum of any kind, it was astounding that he should have remembered my own trivial case at all.

Day after day went by, and still the stream of visitors continued to flow on; as fast as a room was vacated it was again occupied. The two village inns afforded but little accommodation for strangers, so all the peasant houses were called into requisition, and above six hundred people found room in that small place. The peasants do not venture to invest much money in furnishing their rooms more comfortably, for, as one of them said to me, "The moment our Herr Pfarrer dies all will come to an end. He ought only to be forty years old. That would be the thing."

Some enterprising individual was willing to run the risk of building a large house in which to lodge strangers, but I am told that Pfarrer Kneipp laid his veto on the plan, saying that whatever money was brought into the place should benefit his parishioners. For in the midst of all this work, and his, I may say, daily growing European celebrity, the good Pfarrer does not for one moment lose sight of his real work, and is indefatigable in all the branches of his ministry. How he finds time for everything is simply a marvel. I should say he sees at least two hundred patients daily. He told me himself he was obliged to say his mass at a very early hour, as after daylight he was never safe from interruption, and he hardly knew when to find time to read his breviary. My conscience often smote me when, on coming into his room early in the morning, I would find him occupied with it; but, provoking as the interruption must have been, he never once accepted my offer of postponing the consultation. Soon after 7 A.M. the regular stream of patients arrived, and till 10, as a rule, there was not one moment's pause in the succession of people whom he saw. At that hour he would leave his house to go over to the neighbouring convent, an old community of Dominican nuns, which is entirely under his direction and care. Numbers of priests congregate in Wörishofen. Some of these whose health was very seriously impaired, lodged in this convent, and all of them, monks and others, would assemble there for their meals and social intercourse. To these the Pfarrer would now devote himself, and here he was supposed to be invisible to his other patients, except during two hours in the afternoon. His kind heart, however, cannot resist any appeal made to it, and more than one interview in the cloisters count amongst my most agreeable recollections of him. The priests dined at the primitive hour of half-past eleven, and the Pfarrer was supposed to share their meal, but even for this he barely allowed himself a quarter of an hour. A written notice was put up in the *Pfarrhof* that after three o'clock no more visitors were received. This was, however, merely an empty form, and till dusk one patient succeeded another, the only interruption being when he was called away to visit some sick parishioner, or when he went to administer with his own hands the douche or *Guss* to some patient whose case was particularly critical. His only recreation seemed to be his evening walk through the village, when he was usually accompanied by one or two doctors, with whom he would visit some of the most interesting cases. His tall commanding figure, easily recognisable at a distance, was like a landmark seen from far. A small white Pomeranian dog called Spitz was his inseparable companion—so devotedly attached to its master that it could with difficulty be restrained from following him into church, and taking active part in the service. Once or twice, during my stay at Wörishofen, the animal made its escape from the *Pfarrhof*, and came galloping up the aisle, with a ludicrous air of canine triumph, just as the Pfarrer was about to commence his sermon, to the considerable disturbance of the congregation.

Another companion, seen frequently by the Curé's side, was his little niece, to whom he is quite devoted; a magnificently healthy child, always barefoot and bareheaded, and who, if such had been required, would have acted as a splendid advertisement of Pfarrer Kneipp's system.

There is a marked difference between the way in which Pfarrer Kneipp sets to work to attack illness and that to which one is accustomed from doctors in general. In the first place, his attention is principally directed to the state of the circulation, and then he seldom attacks the local evil, but sets to work to strengthen the whole system. In many cases he presses nature into his service, and forces the hitherto hidden evil to appear on the surface.

It is evident that in Germany, at least, Pfarrer Kneipp's cure is going to influence the present state of medicine to a considerable extent. The cures he has effected are too numerous and too striking to pass unnoticed. According to Bavarian law, nothing can be done to prevent him carrying on his treatment as long as he uses no secret remedies—*Geheim-mittel;* and this, indeed, he does not, for he is only too anxious that the public in general, and doctors in particular, should make themselves familiar with the whole matter. At first doctors seemed inclined to pooh-pooh the whole thing, and to smile compassionately when his name was mentioned. This era, however, is past, and their curiosity is evidently aroused. Some men with leading names have, I hear, been honest and sensible enough to send patients whom they could not cure to Wörishofen, whilst a good many, especially younger men, come to study the whole thing for themselves at headquarters. To these the Pfarrer is most courteous, and gives them every opportunity of studying his system and profiting by his experience. Whilst I was there I frequently talked about the whole process with a very intelligent young doctor, who told me frankly that he was quite dumfoundered during the first week of his stay at Wörishofen, as the good Pfarrer simply overthrew most existing theories; "but," said the doctor, "he gives a good reason for every step he takes, and after the cures I see, I am determined to go in for this system myself." He added, that in five weeks at Wörishofen he had learnt more than in his whole university career. The Pfarrer himself says—as he well may, being sixty-nine years of age—that he would only be too thankful to rest and to see others carry on his work. From all I have seen, I think the whole system of this treatment would be admirably in its place in England, where in country parts it is often a great difficulty and expense to find a good doctor. The putting together and dispensing of these simple remedies would also, it seems to me, be a most welcome and interesting occupation to numbers of ladies in the country who devote so great a part of their lives to looking after the poor.

During the nine weeks which at two different intervals I spent there in the summer of 1889,[1] I took care to question many of the other patients about the cures effected, and certainly some were most striking. It was very evident that a great number of the patients who assembled there had sought in vain for help from doctors, and many, as I know, came, having had their death-warrant, so to say, signed. Far from being intimidated by such cases, the Pfarrer openly said he undertook these in preference to others; and if I were to describe all which came directly under my notice, I could write pages. On the same day on which I reached the village, a lad of ten to twelve years was brought there suffering from some complaint of the knee, which, as the doctor declared, rendered amputation necessary. Before I left, at the end of a month, I saw this same boy able to play about with the village urchins, the healthy colour in his cheeks contrasting vividly with the striking pallor they had borne on his arrival. One patient, a Baron S——, suffering from disease of the spinal marrow and pronounced incurable, had to be wheeled in a bath-chair when he arrived at Wörishofen. The Pfarrer at once told him that by the end of a fortnight he would be on his feet again, and this actually came true. Naturally, however, as charity begins at home, I was most drawn to the whole thing by the marvellous effect it had upon myself. Not only was the root of the evil discovered, but the most distressing symptoms

[1] It was during my second visit to Wörishofen that Pfarrer Kneipp himself first suggested to me the idea of translating his book into English, which permission he subsequently ratified and confirmed by a signed document.—Translator's note.

were removed; and I was entirely restored to health in the course of a few months—in fact, regenerated, as the Pfarrer calls it. To return to other cases, I will only name a few to show how very varied they are. Just before I came, a child of eleven had been brought there, cased up in an iron frame, with a distorted hip, and utterly unable to walk. This child had been under the treatment of one of the most celebrated surgeons in Germany, who had failed to cure it. From the first moment the Pfarrer was certain of his success in the case. He is one of the most genial of men and thoroughly enjoys a little joke, so he laid a wager with a gentleman who was present when the child was brought, that in three weeks' time it would come on foot through the village to his house. Just as he had said, three weeks later the child actually walked through the village accompanied by a crowd of people. I repeatedly visited it myself and learnt the full details of this case. Another cure which took place whilst I was there, was one of a man who had completely lost his voice, and who could only speak in a hoarse whisper. He had quite recovered it before I left. In the railway carriage I entered into conversation with a priest, who told me that for a couple of years he had been such an invalid that he had had to give up his parish. All the doctors he consulted agreed that he was suffering from heart-disease, though they differed as to what name to give it. At the first glance the Pfarrer decreed it was not heart-disease, and at the end of a fortnight the patient was able to leave, feeling much better. One priest I heard of recovered his memory, which he had lost from overwork, in the course of three weeks. I must here lay especial stress upon the effect the treatment seems to have on the mental powers.

Whilst the cure itself lasts, one is almost unfit for mental exertion. Even the simple writing of a letter was to me a thing to be dreaded; but a certain stage once past, and the cure reduced to a much lighter degree, as it always is for home use, then it is that one begins to feel its wonderful effects. I am perfectly sure that this cure, consistently carried out in fresh surroundings, might well mean a new lease of working capacity to many a man working hard and straining his mental powers to the utmost.

Pfarrer Kneipp—as he himself says—might be a very rich man by this time if he had chosen to accept what is offered to him, instead of which we find him living in the utmost simplicity of surroundings, deriving no personal benefit from the exercise of his powers. He regards the matter from a higher point of view, as even his enemies are forced to concede, considering his gift as one which he is bound to employ to his best ability for the relief of humanity. In business matters he is innocent as a child, the fees he accepts being barely sufficient to keep him from being an actual loser by his charity.

My own bill for his medical advice during a period of five weeks amounted to the gigantic sum of ten marks; while a gentleman of my acquaintance was charged only six marks for a course of treatment extending over two months.

It is now two years since I last visited Wörishofen, and even this short time has, I am told, wrought considerable changes there. The press of visitors has now become so great that Pfarrer Kneipp has been forced to introduce a certain amount of method into his arrangements in place of the pleasant haphazard manner in which business was formerly conducted. At his mid-day consultations, which take place at the Dominican convent, numbered tickets are now distributed to establish the order of precedence, according to which people are then admitted to his presence in batches of from five to ten simultaneously. It is becoming more and more difficult, I hear, to secure a *tête-à-tête* interview.

A further innovation is the little recipe-books now sold at Wörishofen, containing accurate directions as to the rules and system of the establishment. Numerous selling booths are beginning to start up, in order to meet some of the requirements of the daily increasing visitors, bearing such sign-boards as the following: "Honey and swimming trousers," "Pfarrer Kneipp coffee and cigars," "Pfarrer Kneipp bread and linen."

Nor is now wanting at Wörishofen the inevitable photographer, never tardy in making his appearance upon the scene of any new *Curort;* and patients are thus now enabled to gratify their friends at a distance by a gift of their portrait taken in the fascinating attitude demanded by the *Oberguss,* or else walking barefoot in wet grass with a pair of boots held carelessly in the hand.

Miniature facsimiles of the humble tin watering-can with which the ablutions are mostly performed, are now fabricated in gold or silver to be worn as brooches or suspended as *breloques* to the watch-chain, an invention due to the genius of an enterprising goldsmith in the neighbouring town of N——, who not long since led to the altar a niece and former assistant of Pfarrer Kneipp.

Over a thousand strangers have been simultaneously at Wörishofen throughout this summer, many of them being forced to seek quarters at neighbouring villages. The trains bring likewise scores of daily visitors from Munich or elsewhere, come hither merely for the purpose of a few minutes' consultation, to depart as soon again.

The most remarkable of the guests who have recently visited Wörishofen is Baron Nathaniel Rothschild, who arrived there in the first week of October 1890, accompanied by a cook, a secretary, and two servants. Not finding suitable quarters at Wörishofen, Baron Rothschild lived and slept in his own private saloon carriage at the railway station of Türkheim, about four English miles distant from Wörishofen. He daily repaired to the village for the purpose of taking his *Güsse,* administered by Pfarrer Kneipp himself, who surely must have reckoned among the proudest moments of his sacerdotal ministry these unprecedented opportunities of pouring water over such a distinguished son of Israel!

Barefooted and bareheaded, Baron Rothschild was seen promenading every evening in a meadow near the railway station, to the wondering admiration of the gaping crowd of *Curgäste* who daily enjoyed this quite abnormal spectacle of Crœsus *sans bottes!*

In conclusion, we shall only mention that the resources of Wörishofen having now become wholly inadequate to receive and provide for the ever-increasing conflux of visitors, numerous other hydropathic establishments, organised upon Pfarrer Kneipp's system, have been recently formed both in Germany and Austria, and that up to the present date (August 1891) no fewer than thirty editions of the German work, 'Meine Wasserkur,' have been issued.

These figures and statistics require no further commentary as to the power of the man who, without effort, and almost against his will, has thus rapidly achieved European fame—a power neither to be denied by his detractors, nor explained away on the score of fashion or magnetic influence. Pfarrer Kneipp is neither a genius nor a magician, but a simple man of the people, whose natural gifts and shrewd insight into human nature have been matured and developed by the patient toil of half a century.

A. DE F.

SALZBURG, *August* 1891.

INTRODUCTION.

No two leaves of a tree are absolutely alike; still less does the fate of any one human being resemble that of another, and were each of us before death to write down the history of our life, there would be as many different biographies as there are individuals. Intricate and involved are the paths which in life cross and recross each other, sometimes resembling an inextricable tangle, of which the threads are interwoven seemingly without plan or purpose. So at least it appears to our short-sighted vision, but it is not so in reality. The beacon of faith throws its illuminating rays into this dark chaos, showing how all these intricate paths have been designed from the outset by an all-wise Creator to lead us to a fixed and determined goal. Wonderful, indeed, are the ways of Providence!

When, from the watch-tower of old age, I look down upon the bygone years, and behold the intricate windings of my paths, I observe how these have sometimes run apparently on the very edge of a precipice, only, however, to reissue thence, and conduct me against all hope to the sunny heights of my vocation; and I have every reason to extol the wise and loving dispensation of Providence, the more so as the road which, judged by human lights alone, seemed destined to lead me to a pernicious and certain death, has proved to be a source of renewed life to myself as to countless others.

I was over twenty-one years of age when, with my Wanderbuch [1] in my pocket, I left my home. This document described me as a weaver apprentice; but, since my childhood, something very different had been inscribed on the leaves of my heart. With unspeakable pain and longing for the realisation of my ideal, I had waited long, long years for this discharge: I wished to become a priest. So I went forth into the world, not, as my friends desired and hoped, to wield the shuttle, but to hurry from place to place, seeking for some one willing and able to assist me in my studies.

At this juncture I was befriended by a prelate, now deceased, Mathias Merkle by name, then chaplain at Grönenbach. For two years he instructed and prepared me with such assiduous zeal, that at the end of that time I was able to enter the Gymnasium. The work was not easy, and to all appearance fruitless. After five years of the greatest efforts and privations, I was morally and physically broken down.

On one occasion when my father came to fetch me home from the town for my vacations, we halted at an inn, and there still ring in my ears the words spoken to him by the landlord: "Weaver," he said to him,

[1] Police-book serving as passport to travelling journeymen.

"you are fetching the student for the last time." Nor was the landlord the only man who spoke thus.

At that time we had in our town a military doctor of considerable repute, and well known for his kindness towards poor invalids. In the last two years of my school-time he visited me about two hundred times. Gladly would he have helped me, but his medical art and self-sacrificing charity were baffled by the steadily increasing disease. I myself had long since abandoned all hope, and awaited my end with mute resignation.

I was fond of dipping into books to amuse and distract my thoughts. Chance—I make use of this common expression, vague and unmeaning though it be, for there is no such thing as chance—threw an insignificant little volume in my way. I opened it: it was a treatise on cold-water cure. I turned over its leaves and read there incredible things. Who knows—shot through my brain—who knows whether you will not find your own case within these pages? I searched on and on, till at last every symptom there described tallied and agreed with mine. What joy! what consolation! New hope electrified the exhausted body and the yet more exhausted mind. This little book was the first straw at which I grasped; soon it became the staff on which the patient could lean; to-day I regard it as the lifeboat sent by a merciful Providence in the hour of my greatest need.

This little book, treating of the healing power of cold water, is written by a doctor: its prescriptions are mostly exceedingly violent and severe. I tried them for a quarter of a year, for half a year: I experienced no perceptible improvement, but also no bad effects. This gave me courage. Then came the winter of the year 1849. I was again at Dillingen. Two or three times a-week I sought out a lonely spot, and bathed for some minutes in the Danube. Rapidly I hurried to the bathing-place, more rapidly yet I hurried home to the warm room. I never derived any harm from these cold exercises, but also, as I deemed, small benefit. In the year 1850 I entered the Georginum[1] at Munich. There I found a poor student whose plight was even worse than my own. The doctor of the establishment refused him the health-certificate indispensable for his admission to holy orders, because—so ran the verdict—he had not much longer to live. I had now a dear companion. I initiated him into the mysteries of my little book, whose maxims we set about practising with cheerful rivalry. Before long my friend received the coveted certificate, and is still alive. I myself grew daily stronger, became a priest, and have now exercised my holy functions for over thirty years. My friends are good enough to flatter me by saying that even now, at the age of over sixty-eight, they admire the strength of my voice and the vigour of my body. Water remained my best friend; who can wonder, therefore, if on my side I feel for it the truest friendship?

Those only who have been in want and misery themselves can appreciate the misery of others. The number of suffering people I met with, and the yet greater number and variety of their complaints, incited me to extend my cold-water experiments and to perfect my system of cure. To my first counsellor in the science of cold-water cure, the aforementioned little volume, I owe much heartfelt thanks. Soon, however, I recog-

[1] A seminary for theological students.

nised that the system, such as it was here recommended, required modification. The applications it enjoined were often too rough, too violent, for the human constitution. Such exaggerated treatment only serves to bring the cold-water cure into discredit, and to reinforce the ranks of those who blindly condemn whatever they do not, or but imperfectly, understand.

I must here observe that I do not approve of all the modes of cold-water application at present in use in hydropathic establishments—many of them, in fact, I decidedly condemn—partly on account of their violence, partly because of their one-sidedness. Patients are too often treated in a stereotyped general fashion; and far too little stress is laid on the peculiarities of each separate case. To discriminate, therefore, which applications are adapted to the disease in question, and furthermore to determine how these are to be varied according to the constitution of the patient, is the touchstone of the true physician.

Most emphatically I warn all against too violent, or too frequent, application of cold water, which can only have the result of transforming this healing element into an agent of destruction, and changing the patient's confidence into terror and disgust.

During thirty years I have studied and tested every single application upon my own person. I frankly acknowledge that at three repeated intervals I was obliged to remodel my system and relax the treatment from severity to mildness, and thence to greater mildness still.

The first and third parts of this little work treat of the form in which I make use of water as a healing power. Whilst the former explains and describes the different modes of application, the latter details some special cases to serve as examples.

In the second part (the introduction to which should be carefully read) I have endeavoured to collect, for the benefit of country people, the directions for forming a small household pharmacy.

To each new patient who comes to consult me I address certain questions, in order to avoid the danger of prescribing hastily and without sufficient knowledge. To answer the following questions is likewise the object of this book:—

1. *What is illness? and from what common source do all illnesses proceed?*

The marvellous harmony in the construction of the human frame must be admitted by all. Even the most unbelieving physician, whose lancet and dissecting-knife have failed to detect the seat of the soul, cannot refuse his admiration to the Creator's masterpiece. Man external and internal sings but one song of glorification. "Let everything on me and in me praise the name of the Lord!" This beautiful harmony and order, which we call health, may be upset and disturbed by various interruptions, which we designate by the name of illness. Illnesses, external and internal, belong to man's daily bread, of which he must partake, whether he will or no.

All these diseases, whatever be their name, have, we maintain, their origin, their root, in the blood, or rather in the derangement of the blood, whether this be owing to irregular and imperfect circulation, or else to the presence of poisonous and vicious elements. The network of veins traversing the human frame can be compared to a well-organised system of irrigation. They conduct the sap of life throughout the body, and nourish each part, each organ, in the manner most suitable to its functions. Perfect order, however, can only lie in the right measure and pace. Whatever is too much or too little in the process of circulation disturbs the equilibrium, the harmony of the whole, causes dissension in the parts, puts sickness in the place of health.

2. *How is the cure effected?*

By the tracks left in the snow the practised hunter recognises the nature of the game he follows. These tracks he pursues would he hunt the stag, chamois, or fox. The experienced doctor quickly perceives where the illness lies, its origin and extension. The disease is recognised by its symptoms, and points out to him the course of remedies to be selected. A simple enough process, many will say. This is sometimes so, but not always. If a person comes to me with frost-bitten ears, without difficulty I recognise this to have been caused by cold; and if a man sitting by a millstone suddenly cries out in pain because of his bruised finger, I shall not require to ask him what is the matter? A far less easy question it is, however, to deal with an ordinary headache or with any ailments of the heart, stomach, or nerves. Just as a tiny straw will suffice to impede a large clock in its progress, so the smallest trifle is capable of producing painful disorder in the action of the heart. To discover this trifle is the doctor's task, frequently a very difficult and laborious process, subject to manifold errors and deceptions. Examples of this will be found in the third part of this book.

If I strike the stem of a young oak-tree with an axe, or only with my foot, it will vibrate throughout; each branch will tremble and each leaf be stirred. How false would be my conclusion were I to deduce that because the leaf trembles it must be attacked! No; the leaf but trembles as a natural consequence of the blow the stem has received. Our nerves may be likened to the branches of a tree. How often we hear the expression, "He is suffering from a nervous complaint—his nerves are affected"! What does this mean? Nothing in reality: it is the whole constitution, which, having received a shock, has caused the nerves to vibrate in sympathy.

If with a pair of scissors you carefully cut through the outer rim of a spider's web, the whole net collapses, and this little work of art, composed of such accurately executed circles and triangles, will present but a confused tangle. How mistaken would I be were I thence to infer the spider to have been at fault, and to have woven her silken trap carelessly and incorrectly! It needs but to replace that one little thread, and the previous beautiful harmony is immediately restored! Thus to find and replace the one little thread—here lies the secret of the doctor's art.

3. *In what manner does water effect the cure?*

You can quickly remove an ink-stain from your hand, or cleanse a bleeding wound, by the application of water. How refreshing it is in summer, at the close of a hard day's labour, to wash the sweat from your brow! You feel revived and strengthened. If a mother perceives an incrustation of scurf on her infant's head, she takes warm water and washes it off.

To dissolve, remove, and strengthen: there, then, are the three principal attributes of water; and we maintain water to be capable of curing every curable disease, as its various applications, properly applied, directly attack the root of the evil and have the result—

(*a*) Of dissolving the germs of diseased matter contained in the blood!

(*b*) Of withdrawing the diseased matter from the system.

(*c*) Of restoring the purified blood to its proper state of circulation.

(*d*) Of bracing the weakened constitution, and rendering it fit for renewed exertion.

4. *Whence proceeds the susceptibility of the present generation? Why is it so liable to be attacked by every possible form of disease, many of which were formerly unknown to us even by name?*

Many persons will deem this question superfluous, yet it seems to me one of the greatest importance, and I do not hesitate to affirm that these evils mostly proceed from insufficient hardening and bracing of the system. The effeminacy and degeneration of men have reached a very high pitch. Weakened and weaklings, bloodless and nervous individuals, sufferers from the heart or the digestion, are now almost the rule: the strong and vigorous have become the exception. We are keenly susceptible to every change of weather: the transition from one season to another cannot be accomplished without the accompaniment of colds and catarrhs; in many cases the mere rapid passage from the open air into a warm room cannot be braved with impunity. The state of things was very different forty or fifty years ago; and what is to be the end of all this, if, as we hear daily repeated on all sides, decay begins to set in before the full zenith of strength has been reached? It is surely high time to look these facts in the face.

The best means to employ with a view to hardening and bracing the general system are briefly indicated further on. Equally important chapters might be written upon the subject of diet, dress, and ventilation —but of these we shall treat perhaps another time.[1] I am well aware that my peculiar views will meet with great opposition, yet I cling to them steadfastly, for they have been ripened and developed by long years of experience and practice. These are no mushroom thoughts which have sprung up overnight in my brain, but true fruits whose savour may be acid or bitter at first taste, but whose beneficial effects will be recognised by all who have tried them.

I will merely here indicate, with regard to food, that what I principally advocate is a dry, simple, nourishing diet, free from all spices and condiments; and as beverage, the pure crystal element which the Creator has so lavishly provided for His creatures. At the same time I am no Puritan, and do not lay my veto upon a glass of wine or beer, but do not attach much importance to their use. From a medicinal point of view, as for instance for convalescents, these stimulating beverages may sometimes be useful: for those in health I consider ripe fruit to be far more advantageous.

[1] See the author's second work, entitled 'So sollt Ihr leben.' Josef Kösel, Kempten, Bayern.

With regard to dress I cling to the old adage—

> "Home made and home spun
> Is the best for every one."

I am particularly opposed to the unequal mode of dress which generally prevails, more especially in winter. The head has its fur cap, the throat a tight collar over which is wrapped a heavy comforter, the shoulders bear a three or four fold covering, to which is added a further wrap, sometimes a fur, for going out of doors. The poor neglected feet alone are covered as in summer by socks or stockings, shoes or boots. What is the result of this senseless partiality? As a pump draws up the water, so the blood rises to the head, the lower extremities become bloodless and cold. Headaches, congestions, distensions of the head veins are the unavoidable consequences. I furthermore disapprove of flannel or wool in any shape coming in direct contact with the skin, and recommend in preference a firm dry simple make of pure home-spun linen. Wool, in my opinion, only tends to absorb heat and sap from the body, aggravating the poverty of blood of our weak nerveless generation.

I will now speak of ventilation. We give the preference to fish which have their origin in pure springs, or, better still, in mountain torrents. The inhabitants of lowland streams and rivers have already less value, and those found in bogs and swamps are utterly to be rejected. In like manner we may speak of a bog-like or swampy atmosphere, and those who breathe it are nourishing their lungs with a pestilential element. The air inhaled for the third time is directly poisonous, has said a celebrated doctor. How many illnesses might be avoided if people would only comprehend of what importance it is to provide for good healthy unadulterated air in their rooms, more especially in their sleeping apartments!

Too great a degree of warmth is likewise injurious to the health. In an overheated room the air is deteriorated, the pure oxygen being thereby destroyed, and the atmosphere rendered unfit for the use of human lungs. 12° to 14° of Réaumur (59° to 64° Fahr.) are amply sufficient, and no room should ever be heated beyond 15° R. (66° Fahr.). Let every one daily see to the thorough and consistent ventilation of all dwelling and sleeping apartments. Of special importance it is that the beds should be thoroughly aired.

I have now said what I had to say at this stage. The preceding will have sufficed to show the portrait of this stranger, who knocks at your door, dear reader; for you it is to decide whether you will say "Come in," or bid him go further. I am prepared for both modes of reception, and declare myself to be satisfied with either.

PART I.

COLD-WATER APPLICATIONS.

"Aquæ omnes . . . laudent nomen Domini."

GENERAL OBSERVATIONS.

STARTING from the presumption that all diseases having their seat in the blood are to be traced either to the presence therein of unwholesome matter, or else to defective or irregular circulation, our cold-water applications pursue a threefold object, viz. :—

1. To dissolve the poisonous germs contained in the blood.
2. To withdraw all unhealthy matter from the system.
3. To strengthen and brace the constitution.

In a general way it may be assumed that the first result is to be achieved by means of fomentations and warm baths infused with herbs. For the second, it will be necessary chiefly to employ various wrappers, assisted according to expediency by compresses and affusions; while the third condition of hardening and bracing the system will best be accomplished by means of cold baths, affusions, lavations, and other means to be indicated hereafter.

The true and rational water-lover—such as I understand him to be—will never fall into the error of seeking for personal satisfaction in the choice of his remedies. Neither will he make a boast of having undergone a certain number of fomentations, affusions, and compresses, nor obstinately cling to any particular application which happens to be congenial. Whenever a result can be obtained with slight means, it were folly to employ stronger ones. This remark is no casual one; for nothing brings cold water into such discredit, as a sanitary and healing power, as the indiscreet, exaggerated, and senseless manipulation of some people.

A few more general observations with regard to the manner in which the cold-water applications are to be employed, may here find place.

Most of these are accomplished by means of cold water, and unless it be directly specified to the contrary, the expression "water" throughout this work is to be taken to signify "cold water." The colder the better is the motto which experience has taught me to cling to; and for healthy persons, an admixture of snow in the water employed for their affusions in winter is highly to be recommended.

To beginners in the water-cure, more especially the aged and the very young, weak and nervous persons who shrink from the cold, as well as those who from nature possess but little latent heat, I frequently permit the use of water which has been warmed to 64° to 66° Fahr., until they can be gradually accustomed to a lower temperature.

The warm applications are in each case minutely described, accurate direction being given with regard to temperature and duration.

With regard to the cold-water applications, we have still a few words to say in order to regulate the patient's conduct before, during, and after these exercises.

No one who feels chilly should attempt to make use of a cold-water application, unless this be directly specified. The application must be performed as rapidly as possible (though without anxiety or slovenly haste), and no unnecessary time should be lost in dressing and undressing. Practical persons will understand so to arrange their costume as to dispense as much as possible with buttons, strings, &c. A cold plunge-bath, for instance, may be accomplished —inclusive of undressing and dressing—in the space of five minutes. A very little practice will enable any one to do this. Whenever an application is directed to be used for the space of one minute, this indicates the shortest term. When, however, it is marked from two to three minutes, the latter space should never be exceeded. To country people, who either possess no pocket-watch, or else are upon distant terms with their timepieces, I usually prescribe the simpler method of counting each minute by means of reciting two Paternosters.

In no case, the head and hands alone excepted, is it permissible to dry the body after an application. The dry clothes are to be replaced on the wet body as quickly as possible, after which the patient is to walk or take other active exercise until the body be completely dry, and has regained its normal temperature. The movement should at first be faster, then slackened gradually. Overheating should, however, be avoided, and those persons whose nature inclines to profuse perspiration should walk slower and for a longer period than less plethoric ones.

As a general rule, it may be assumed that a quarter of an hour's exercise after each application is the minimum, which should never be curtailed.

Neither friction nor rubbing has any place in my system; their first object—that of restoring warmth to the body—being far better and more equally achieved by the simpler plan of not drying; while the action of the coarse linen shirt upon the damp skin fulfils the second condition of opening the pores and restoring activity to the epidermis—having, moreover, the further advantage of keeping up a constant gentle friction by night and by day, without waste of time or trouble.

As a final observation, I must call attention to the fact that cold-water applications taken in the evening are apt to disagree with some people, by unduly exciting the nervous system and causing restless or disturbed sleep; with others, on the contrary, the effect is a diametrically opposite one. It is therefore of great importance that each person should carefully study and ascertain their individualities on this as on other points.

APPLIANCES FOR HARDENING AND BRACING THE SYSTEM.

These may be enumerated as follows:—

1. Walking barefoot—
   (*a*) In wet grass.
   (*b*) On wet stones.
   (*c*) In fresh-fallen snow.
   (*d*) In cold water.
2. Foot-baths and arm-baths.
3. Knee affusions—either with or without the accompaniment of upper and lower affusions.

1. The simplest and most natural practice for bracing the system is *walking barefoot.*

This can be practised and varied in manifold ways, so as to meet the requirements of age, sex, and condition.

Quite little children, who are still dependent on the help of others and mostly confined to the room or to swaddling-clothes, should never wear any foot-covering of whatever kind. If only I could sufficiently impress this important rule on the minds of all parents!

Instinct usually comes to the help of those children

who are able to stand or move about. Gleefully they tear off their heavy uncomfortable feet-coverings, happy to be able to disport themselves unshackled and free. The children of the poor are rarely interfered with in this self-assertion of nature, but the offspring of wealthy parents are less fortunate; and even when the parents are sufficiently sensible to perceive the advantages of this mode of bringing up, there are many impediments. In large towns people cannot walk about barefoot without attracting attention, and not every one is lucky enough to possess a secluded garden, where such exercises may be practised unnoticed. In default of this, however, it will not be difficult for parents to organise that at certain hours of the day the children should be made to take regular barefooted exercise in a room or corridor.

(*a*) Particularly effective is the *barefooted walking in wet grass*, whether the moisture be produced by dew, rain, or artificial means.

The wetter the grass, and the more this exercise be prolonged and repeated, the greater will be its results. As a rule, the grass-walking may extend from one to three quarters of an hour. Attention must be paid to keeping shoes and stockings dry; for if, as imprudent young persons are sometimes apt to do, these have been carelessly tossed aside in the wet grass and allowed to absorb moisture, the beneficial effects of the exercise will be counteracted.

(*b*) Where grass is not available, *walking barefooted on wet stones* may be made to serve the same purpose. There are few houses where a stone-flagged corridor or brick-laid kitchen-floor is not to be found, a portion of which can be moistened by means of a watering-can, which proceeding is to be repeated as soon as the moisture begins to evaporate. For persons who practise this exercise as a remedy, a period of from three to fifteen minutes should not be exceeded. Healthy people, who practise it simply with a view to bracing the system, may, however, extend their walk to half an hour and even longer.

Whoever is subject to cold feet, throat affections, catarrhs, headaches, and congestions, should often employ this remedy. A little vinegar mixed with the water will render it still more efficacious.

(*c*) Of more powerful effect than the two aforenamed practices, is the *walking barefooted in new-fallen snow,* which is soft and powdery, or else in snow which, beginning to thaw, is in a soft slushy state. Old congealed snow, which has lain for several days and become stiff and hard, is, however, unfit for this purpose. It is likewise undesirable to perform this exercise when there is a cold wind. A little self-control will be required to take the first few steps, but a pleasant reaction will quickly follow. I am acquainted with persons who are accustomed to prolong these snowy walks for an hour, and even beyond that, with the best results; but as a general rule, from three to four minutes will be sufficient.

So much with regard to snow-walking for the healthy. The following two cases will show how it is often a direct means of cure in certain illnesses.

A person who had suffered from chilblains, which used to suppurate and cause much pain during many years, was advised by me to try snow-walking as a cure. She followed my advice, and was soon perfectly cured of her distressing complaint.

Quite recently a young girl came to me complaining of violent toothache. "If you walk five minutes in the fresh-fallen snow, your toothache will speedily disappear," I said to her. She ran out into the garden and did so, whence she returned some ten minutes later with the joyful announcement that her toothache was completely gone.

(*d*) *Walking in water.*—Simple as it sounds to walk about in water which reaches up to the calf of the

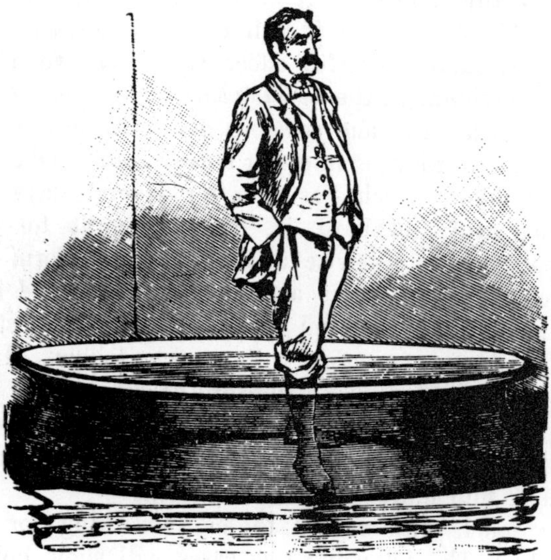

Fig. 1.

leg, this practice is most efficacious, and of direct influence in many diseases which have their seat in the bowels, bladder, and kidneys. It relieves the lungs, expels noxious gas from the stomach, and removes headache. It can be practised in any sort of bath or tub, which should at first contain only sufficient water to reach to the ankle (see fig. 1), the quantity to be increased by degrees, until after a time the whole calf up to the knee is covered: one minute to begin with, which, later on, may be extended to five or six minutes. Weak or nervous persons may employ lukewarm water at first; but for those who can stand it, the colder it is the better, and a slight admixture of snow in winter will render it still more efficacious.

2. A special means of hardening the extremities is the following: After having stood in cold water up to the knees for one minute, shoes and stockings are to be replaced, and the arms, bared to the shoulder, are likewise to be held in water for a similar space of time. Still better it is to perform both these acts simultaneously, which can either be done in one large bath or in two smaller ones. The tub for the arms to be placed on a chair to facilitate the process.

This proceeding is of great use for convalescents after certain illnesses, where it is necessary to increase the circulation of blood at the extremities.

The arms alone may be bathed with advantage by persons suffering from chilblains and cold hands.

3. A last recipe for bracing the system is the *knee affusion*, of which a description will be found later on in this work. The knee affusion is the feet's best friend, as it lures and entices the reluctant blood down into the imperfectly filled veins. This practice may be varied and modified in manifold ways, to be explained hereafter.

The knee affusion should never be employed when

the body is cold or shivering; but cold feet only (if the rest of the body be warm) are no impediment to its use. I must also premise that the knee affusion alone—that is, when not made use of in conjunction with other cold-water applications—should never be continued for more than three to four consecutive days at a time. Those who employ it for a longer period do so mostly in combination and alternation with the upper affusion, or with the arm-bath just described.

All these various practices for strengthening and bracing the system may, with slight variations and modifications, be made use of at any season; in winter some of these may require to be shortened, in contradistinction to which the span of exercise to be taken after each application may be proportionally increased. Novices would do well not to begin their course of hardening in winter, but should rather defer it to a more genial season.

WATER APPLICATIONS.

THE cold-water applications of which I make use may be catalogued under the following heads:- -

(*A*) Compresses.
(*B*) Baths.
(*C*) Vapour baths or steamings.
(*D*) Affusions.
(*E*) Lavations.
(*F*) Swathings.
(*G*) Water-drinking.

(*A*) COMPRESSES.

1. THE UPPER COMPRESS.

A large piece of coarse linen (sackcloth is best for the purpose)—which, when laid together from three to ten fold, should be long and broad enough to cover the entire body from the throat to below the abdomen—is steeped in cold water, well wrung out, and applied to the reclining patient. Over this is drawn a second three or four fold piece of dry linen, or else a woollen blanket, which has the object of excluding the outer air. A cloth or woollen scarf should likewise be placed round the neck.

The compress, which is to be applied from forty-five minutes to an hour, must in many cases be renewed from time to time—that is to say, the linen is to be taken off and dipped again in fresh cold water.

When the prescribed time has elapsed and the compress been removed, the patient should either rise from bed, and, quickly dressing, take exercise, or else remain lying until the body has regained its normal temperature.

The upper compress has specially the effect of expelling unwholesome gases from the stomach and bowels.

2. The Lower Compress.

The lower compress is often used alternately with the upper one, and, like it, is to be taken in bed. To avoid wetting the mattress, a thick woollen rug or blanket should first be spread, and above this the three or four fold wet linen sheet, long enough to cover the whole back from the nape of the neck to the end of the spine. The woollen rug should then be folded upwards over the patient, who is furthermore covered with other blankets or quilts. Like the upper compress, the lower one may also be applied for three-quarters of an hour to an hour, and is to be renewed in like fashion.

Its functions are to strengthen the spine and spine marrow, to cure pains in the back and acute rheumatic affections. Also in cases of fever it is highly efficacious.

3. Upper and Lower Compress conjointly employed.

The two compresses can be applied not only alternately (in which case the lower compress always takes precedence of the upper one), but likewise simultaneously and for the same length of time as previously indicated. In cases of high fever, gases, congestion, and hypochondriasis, these two compresses taken together will be found useful.

4. Compress on the Abdomen.

A four to six fold linen cloth, previously dipped in water, and well wrung out, is applied to the lower part of the patient's body, which must be carefully covered up as in the foregoing applications. It may remain from three-quarters of an hour to two hours, but should be renewed at the end of an hour. This compress will render good service in cases of indigestion, stomach cramp, and whenever it is desirable to draw away the blood from heart or chest.

According to expediency, as hereafter indicated, the water may be mixed with vinegar or various herb decoctions.

(*B*) BATHS.

I. Foot-baths.

Foot-baths may be taken cold or warm.

1. *The Cold Foot-bath*

consists in putting the feet up to or above the calves from one to three minutes.

Its chief effect is to draw down the blood from head and chest. It is, however, mostly employed in combination with other water applications, as in cases where the patient for some reason or other is unable to stand whole or semi baths.

For healthy people it achieves the result of curing fatigue and producing sound wholesome sleep. It cannot be too strongly recommended to country people, especially in summer after a hard day's work.

2. *The Warm Foot-bath*

can be taken in various ways.

(*a*) Put a handful of salt and twice that quantity of wood-ashes into a pail of water, whose temperature should be from 86° to 91° F. Duration of foot-bath from twelve to fifteen minutes.

Occasionally I prescribe a foot-bath with a temperature as high as 100° F., in which case, however, the warm foot-bath is invariably followed by a cold one of half a minute.

Warm foot-baths are chiefly to be recommended to weak, nervous, bloodless individuals, to the very young or very old, and to those of the weaker sex. They will be found effective in case of congestion, head and throat affections, cramps, &c.

(*b*) *The hay-flower foot-bath* is specially strengthening in its effects.

Pour boiling water over a small apronful (three to five handfuls) of hay-flowers—viz., refuse of hay, containing leaves, flowers, grass seed, &c.—cover up the jar or pot, and use as foot-bath as soon as it has sunk to a temperature of 88° to 91° F. It is a matter of indifference whether the flowers are allowed to remain in the water, or have been previously strained away.

These foot-baths are of great and valuable service in many foot-complaints—open wounds, bruises, boils, putrefaction of the toes and suppuration of the nails—likewise in cases where the feet have suffered from tight shoes.

(*c*) *The oat-straw foot-bath* is closely related to the foregoing one.

The straw is boiled for half an hour, and then used as a foot-bath from twenty to thirty minutes, at a temperature of from 88° to 91° F.

Experience has taught me that these foot-baths are invaluable for corns, scirrhous tumours, and suchlike growths. Sometimes they are to be employed in combination with cold foot-baths.

(*d*) *Foot-bath of malt-husks.*

The feet to be placed in a pail containing warm malt-husks without admixture of water, and kept there from fifteen to thirty minutes. Very efficacious in all cases of gout and rheumatism.

An observation to which special importance must be attached is that persons suffering from varicose veins should never take a foot-bath in which the water rises above the ankles: they should also never go beyond a temperature of 88° F.

Foot-baths of simple warm water—that is to say, without other admixture—I never employ nor prescribe.

II. Semi-baths.

By semi-bath I understand those in which the water reaches only to the centre or lower part of the abdomen. They can be made use of in threefold fashion, viz.:—

(*a*) By standing in the water, so that this reaches above the calves or above the knees.

(*b*) By kneeling in the water, so that the thighs are likewise covered.

(*c*) Sitting in the water, which reaches to the pit of the stomach.

All three modes of semi-baths, which are invariably taken with cold water, are chiefly to be classified among the means for hardening and bracing the system, and are therefore more often to be used by the healthy than by invalids. When made use of as a remedy for certain diseases, their application must always be directly specified and explained; made use of at hazard, they frequently do more harm than good. Whether for the healthy or the sick, they never are used except in conjunction with other applications, nor should their duration ever exceed the space of three minutes.

The two first modes of semi-baths—namely, standing and kneeling in the water—are of great use in cases of debility, especially when the patient from various causes is unable to endure the pressure of a complete bath. Taken in combination with the arm-bath, they are most valuable for strengthening and bracing the system.

The third semi-bath is to be recommended to all healthy people without exception, as well as in the manifold diseases of the lower part of the body, whose name is legion.

III. Sitz baths.

The sitz-baths are to be employed either cold or warm.

(*a*) *The cold sitz-bath* is taken in the following manner: In default of the regular sitz-bath, whose shape is familiar to us (*a*, fig. 2), a common low wooden tub (*b*, fig. 2) can be employed.

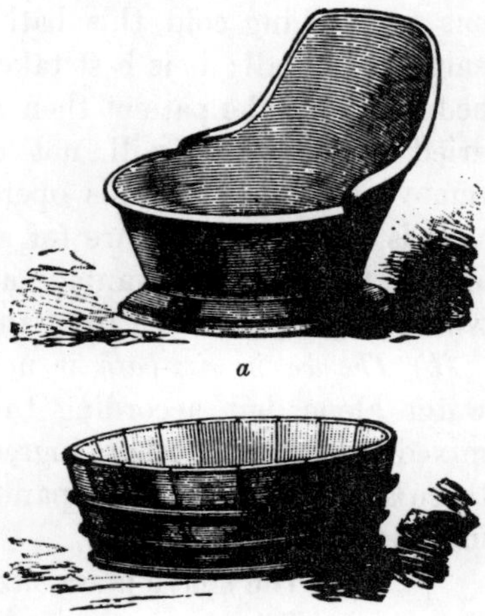

a

b

Fig. 2.

In this bath or tub the patient is seated in such manner that the water covers the upper part of the thigh, and reaches to the middle of the abdomen, the legs from the thigh downwards remaining free (fig. 3).

The duration of the cold sitz-bath is from half a minute to three minutes.

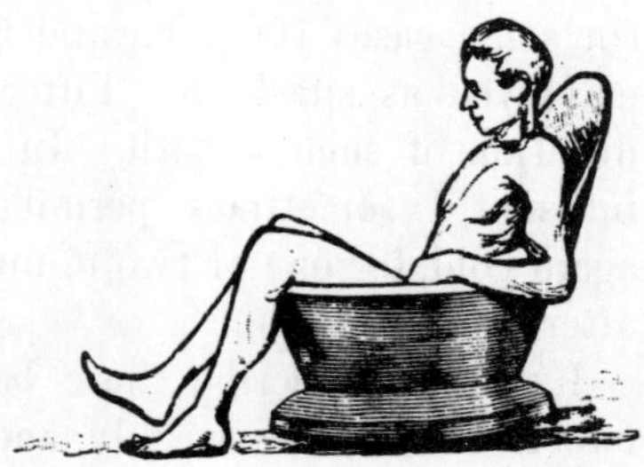

Fig. 3.

The sitz-bath, like the semi-bath, is one of the most valuable and useful among the water applications, second to none in its effects upon the digestion and intestines. It serves to regulate the circulation, to expel unhealthy gases, and is particularly efficacious in cases of chlorosis, bloody flux, and many other like complaints.

To ward off catarrhs and render the system impervious to catching cold, this bath should be frequently employed by all: it is best taken at night, direct from bed, to which the patient then returns without having dried himself. It will not even be necessary to remove the shirt for this operation.

It is an invaluable cure for sleeplessness; and may also be taken with advantage after a bad night's rest when we awake feeling tired and unrefreshed.

(*b*) *The warm sitz-bath* is never prepared of warm water alone, but according to my system is always mixed with some other ingredient. The following three are the principal preparations of which I make use in this form, viz.:—

The shave-grass sitz-bath.
The oat-straw sitz-bath.
The hay-flower sitz-bath.

The preparation of these three baths is identical. The herb is infused in boiling water, after which it is allowed to cool down to a temperature of 86° to 91° (in some cases 100°) F., and then, without straining, employed as sitz-bath. Fifteen minutes is the usual duration of such a bath. In order not to waste the infusion, I sometimes permit it to be made use of again cold, for one or two minutes, three or four hours after the first bath.

I seldom prescribe these baths oftener than from two to three times weekly, and mostly in conjunction with other applications.

The shave-grass sitz-bath is of great service in

diseases of the bladder and kidneys, in gravel and stone complaints.

The oat-straw sitz-bath is excellent for all gouty and rheumatic affections.

The hay-flower sitz-bath is more of general effect, and may be used instead of the two foregoing when these are not to be procured. It has always rendered me good service in cases of boils, constipation, piles, and colic.

IV. Full Baths.

These baths may also be divided into warm and cold baths. Both kinds are made use of for the healthy as well as the sick.

1. *The Cold Full Bath*

can be used in twofold fashion. Either you recline in the bath in such manner that the whole body is covered by the water, or else—in order to avoid the pressure on the lungs for those who dislike it—you sit in the bath with the water reaching only to the armpits. In this latter case the upper chest and neck must be rapidly washed over with a rough towel.

The shortest duration of this bath is half a minute; the longest three minutes. In general, the shorter the bath the more efficacious are its results, and whoever stays one minute only in the full bath is wiser than he who stays five minutes.

(*a*) *Cold Full Baths for the Healthy.*

With regard to these baths the principal questions to be answered are the following:—

In what condition must be the healthy body in order to derive benefit from these cold baths?

How long is it permissible to remain in the cold bath?

In what season is it advisable to begin this course of hardening the system?

The first condition to be observed is that the entire body be warm before entering the cold water. Whoever feels cold or chilly will be unwise in taking a cold bath; but profuse perspiration is no objection to its use, provided it be employed with sense and discrimination.

This leads us to the second question—namely, the duration of such baths. To take a cold full bath, undress quickly and lie down in the water for one minute. If you are in perspiration, then sit in the water till the middle of the chest and rapidly wash over the upper body with a towel or sponge. Having quickly dressed again, take exercise till the body has regained its normal temperature—at least a quarter of an hour. Workmen may return to their occupation if it be of a kind calculated to restore the circulation.

The important task of hardening and bracing the system cannot be begun too soon with a view to warding off disease. It would, however, be highly imprudent to begin at once with extreme measures, and many persons will do well to go through some little course of preparation before embarking in our full baths. (See means of hardening and bracing the system.)

I do not advise any one to take more than three such baths weekly.

(*b*) *Cold Full Bath for Invalids.*

Under the head of diseases I have specified how and when these baths are to be applied in each separate case. A few general remarks may, however, find place here.

A healthy robust constitution is enabled to cast off the germ of illness by its own unaided strength. In sick and weakly bodies this process must be assisted and promoted by carefully selected means.

The cold full bath is one of these means, and may be used with great advantage in all cases of violent fever. More harmless and efficacious by far than the expensive quinine, the cheap antipyrin, the poisonous digitalis, and the many other intoxicating and stupefying drugs, is pure cold water intelligently applied. We have no other means of putting out a fire but by water; and what is fever but an internal conflagration which water alone can cure?

Quite recently, in Austria, the treatment of typhus patients with cold water has been advocated and introduced in some of the military hospitals. This is a step in the right direction; but why should typhus alone be treated in this fashion? Who says A must also be prepared to say B; and the same course equally applies to all diseases in which the temperature is raised to fever-heat.

2. *The Warm Full Bath,*

like the cold, may be used by sick and healthy.

It can be used in twofold fashion: the bather reclines in a bath or tub sufficiently filled with water to cover the entire body (see A, fig. 4), from twenty-five to thirty minutes. Alongside is a second bath filled with cold water (B, fig. 4), into which he then rapidly plunges for one minute only, before resuming his clothes. In default of this second bath, quickly washing over the body with cold water may serve the same purpose. Without drying, the bather resumes his clothes and takes exercise, at least half an hour, until he is thoroughly warm and dry. The

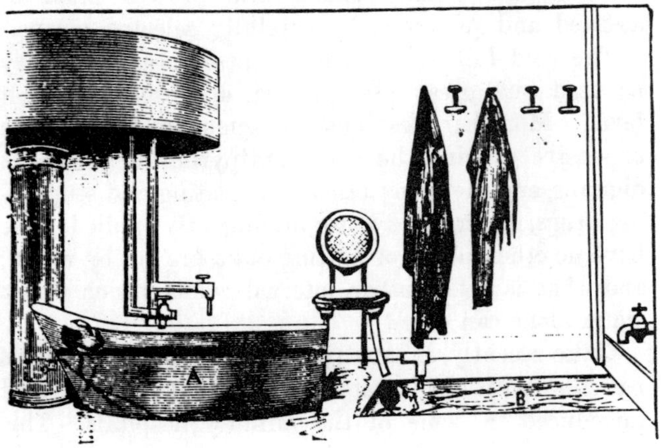

Fig. 4.

temperature of the first bath may be from 91° to 95° F., for the aged from 95° to 100° F.

The second mode of taking this bath is as follows: As in the first instance, the bath is filled with warm water, which, however, must have a temperature of from 100° to 111° F.

This bath is taken not once, but thrice, each time with transition into the cold water. The whole proceeding lasts exactly thirty-three minutes, and is divided as follows:—

Ten minutes in the warm water;
One minute in the cold water.
Ten minutes in the warm water;
One minute in the cold water.
Ten minutes in the warm water;
One minute in the cold-water.

The cold plunge or washing invariably forms the conclusion of the process.

I never order warm baths alone without the sequel of cold-water bath or sponging. Likewise I seldom make use of simple warm baths without the admixture of some herb or grass infusion.

(a) *The Warm Full Bath for the Healthy.*

Under this designation I understand merely the relatively healthy, for thoroughly healthy persons require no warm bath, but should keep to cold water.

Young, weak, and nervous persons may, however, be permitted to take warm baths; likewise women whose strength has been exhausted by their domestic and maternal duties. Such a bath, with a temperature of 95° F., may be taken once a-month, from twenty-five to thirty minutes, always succeeded, however, by a cold plunge or lavation.

(b) *The Warm Full Bath for the Sick.*

These warm baths may be divided into—

Hay-flower baths.
Oat-straw baths.
Pine-needle baths.
Mixed baths.

The preparation of the two first baths has already been explained under the head of Sitz-baths. A few words may, however, be added by way of precaution.

The Hay-flower Bath.—A little bag filled with hay-flowers is thrown into a pot of boiling water, and left there to infuse for at least fifteen minutes. The infusion is then to be mixed with warm or cold water, according to the temperature of the bath to be taken. This bath, the simplest and easiest to prepare, is likewise the most natural and innocent one for restoring warmth to the body. The coffee-hued liquid tends to open the pores and dissolve unwholesome secretions.

The Oat-straw Bath.—When a good bunch of oat-straw has been boiled in a kettle for half an hour, the infusion is to be employed as above.

This bath is more powerful in its workings than the hay-flower bath, and is of great service in all complaints of the bladder and kidneys, as well as in cases of gout, gravel, and stone.

The Pine-tree Bath.—To prepare this, take pine-needles — the fresher the better — small broken-up twigs of the pine-tree, and resinous cones chopped up in small pieces; boil all together half an hour, and use as above. This bath is likewise of much effect on kidneys and bladder, though weaker in its effects than the oat-straw bath. It principally acts upon the skin by restoring activity to the epidermis. It is specially to be recommended to the aged.

Mixed baths is the title I have given to those prepared out of more than one sort of herb. When, for instance, there is not a sufficient quantity of one or other herb at hand, two or three may be mixed. I frequently mix oat-straw with hay-flowers, by boiling these two together.

3. *Mineral Baths.*

A word here as to mineral baths in answer to the many questions which have been addressed to me on the subject.

All mineral baths are directly opposed to my system, because I am a sworn enemy of extreme measures; and just as I never advocate the use of Turkish towels, wire flesh-brushes, and other like drastic measures, so, too, am I no friend of mineral baths. All these waters, whatever be their name, contain more or less pungent salts and acids. We do not employ coarse sand in order to clean delicate gold or silver vessels; and our internal organs are surely not less delicate and precious than these?

V. Partial Baths.

1. *Hand and Arm Baths.*

The title sufficiently indicates the nature of these baths, whose application will be found in the third part of this work.

2. *The Head-bath.*

This bath is one of the most important. It can be taken warm or cold, in the following manner:—

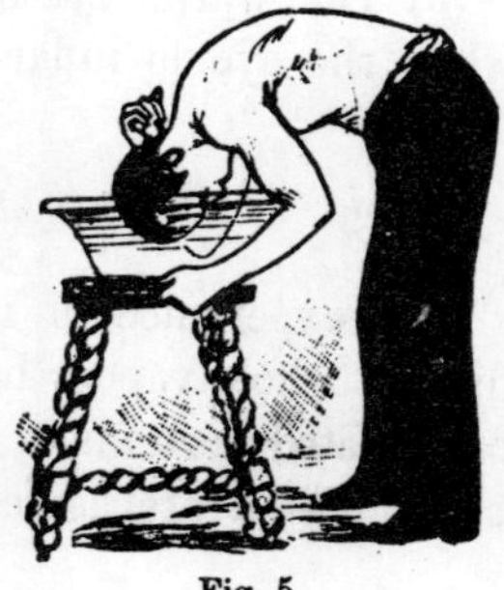

Fig. 5.

Place a small tub or deep basin on a chair, and plunge the upper head in water (see fig. 5) for one minute if the water be cold, from five to seven if warm. Wet the back of the head with the hand, so that all hair down to the nape of the neck be moistened. The hair to be carefully dried after the bath. This is the only case in which drying is permitted, wet hair being conducive to rheumatism.

I frequently prescribe the head-bath in cases of ringworm, dry scab, &c.

3. *The Eye bath,*

which can be taken warm or cold, consists merely in dipping the face with open eyes in a basin of water during half a minute. The process may be repeated as often as four or five times, always with half a minute or a minute's interval between two plunges. The warm eye-bath (86° to 91° F.), which must always terminate with a cold bath, is never prepared of warm water alone, but has invariably an admixture of some herb infusion such as fennel or eyebright.

(*a*) The cold eye-bath is excellent for weak but healthy eyes. It strengthens and revives the inner and outer vessels.

(*b*) The warm eye-bath (lukewarm) is employed when the eye is inflamed or otherwise diseased.

(*C*) VAPOUR BATHS.

The experience of many years has taught me to discard whole vapour baths, and only to employ steam on isolated portions of the body. The applications I make use of are as follows:—

1. The Head Vapour Bath.

For this are requisite a small wooden tub with a tight-fitting lid and two handles on which the arms can lean (fig. 6), two chairs, and a thick woollen blanket. Of the two chairs or stools, the higher one serves to sit upon; on the lower one is placed the tub filled with boiling water. The patient, stripped to the waist, takes his place on the higher chair, and having covered himself tent-fashion with the blanket (fig. 7) and removed the lid of the tub, he leans over it in such a manner that the ascending steam completely envelops his head and upper body.

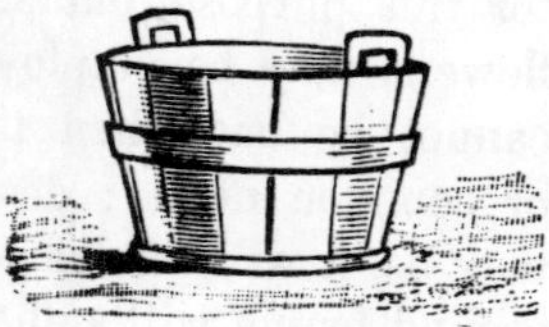

Fig. 6.

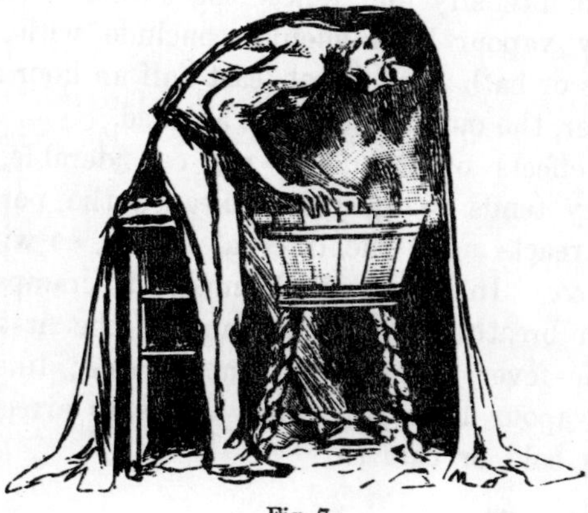

Fig. 7.

This application may last from twenty to twenty-four minutes, at the end of which time the blanket is removed and the whole upper body vigorously sponged with cold water, to be succeeded by exercise either in or out of doors, according to the season.

It must here be remarked that, as pure steam has sometimes an unfavourable effect on the eyes, I never employ it except in combination with some herb infusions. I give the preference to fennel over all others for this purpose, but also mint, sage, elder and lime flowers, may be employed with advantage. If these cannot be had, then take a handful of hay-flowers or common nettle: despised though the latter plant may be, it will render good service. One spoonful of ground fennel will suffice for a single application.

For those to whom perspiration does not come easily, a piece of brick made red-hot on the kitchen fire may be introduced into the tub about ten minutes after the beginning of the vapour bath. This will serve to intensify and renew the steam.

Every vapour bath should conclude with a cold lavation or bath; and for at least half an hour after it, in winter, the outer air is to be avoided.

The effects of this bath are considerable, for it not only tends to open and cleanse the pores, but it also reacts upon the internal organs, as windpipe, lungs, &c. In cases of rheumatism, cramps, difficulty in breathing, headaches, and in the first stages of slime-fever, it renders great service; likewise a single vapour bath will often suffice to arrest a beginning cold or catarrh.

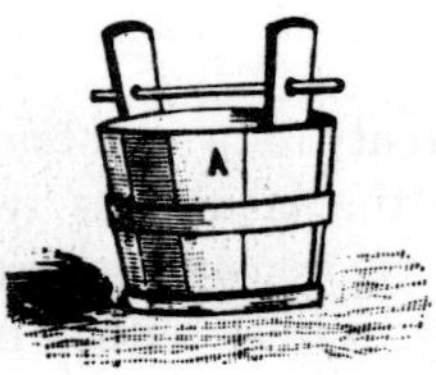

Fig. 8.

2. The Vapour Foot-bath.

As with the upper body, this process may be applied to the lower members.

The application is as follows:—A thick woollen blanket is spread over the chair, on which the patient, having bared feet and legs, takes his place; before him the foot-bath or tub half filled with boiling water (fig. 8), and placed across it from sidé to side a narrow board on which to rest the feet. A little contrivance (fig. 9) will readily enable him to fasten this board securely to avoid the disagreeable feeling of its slipping to and fro. When everything is thus prepared, the blanket is to be wrapped over the front of the legs so as completely to exclude the air (fig. 10).

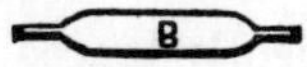

Fig. 9.

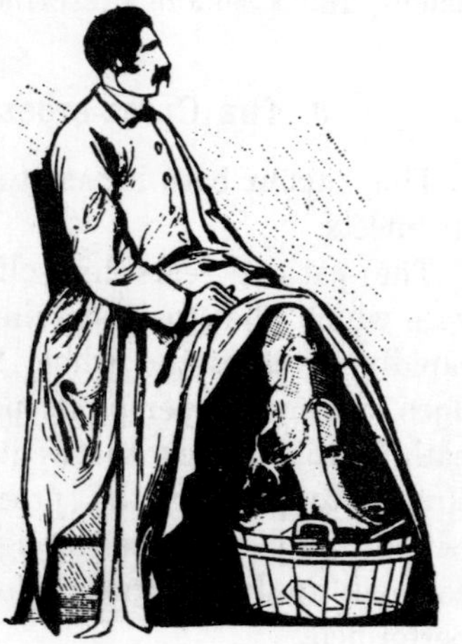
Fig. 10.

For the vapour foot-bath I usually employ a light infusion of hay-flowers, and, as with the upper vapour bath, its effect may be increased after the lapse of ten minutes by the introduction of a piece of red-hot brick into the water. The duration of the foot-bath depends entirely upon the nature of the complaint and the result to be achieved. From fifteen to twenty minutes with one piece of red-hot brick is the mildest form of foot-bath, which may, however, be extended from twenty-five to thirty minutes, while the red-hot brick may be renewed at intervals of from five to ten minutes.

As in the foregoing, the vapour foot-bath must invariably be concluded with a cold ablution.

This bath is employed in many foot complaints, as

also in case of profuse and offensive perspiration. Where there is a threatening of blood-poisoning it is likewise useful, as well as for cramps and congestions of blood to the head.

Weak, bloodless individuals who are not yet sufficiently braced to make use of cold-water applications, have often derived great benefit from these foot-baths.

The vapour foot-bath must not be employed too frequently. One or two weekly of these will usually be sufficient, and I seldom prescribe them as often as thrice.

3. The Close-stool Vapour Bath.

This vapour bath is easy to prepare and excellent in its effects.

The patient seats himself on the chair or metal vase which the stool contains. The ascending steam rapidly envelops the whole body, so as often to produce a general perspiration. The duration of this bath is from fifteen to twenty minutes. If it be desirable to prolong the process of perspiration, the patient may then be brought to bed and warmly covered up for a time before the cold ablution be performed.

The action of this bath is pre-eminently to dissolve and secrete unhealthy matter, which is thus removed by sweating. As in other cases, I never here use warm water alone, but always the aforementioned admixtures of oat-straw, hay-flower, or, best of all, shave-grass.

Oat-straw vapour is employed for diseases of the kidneys and for stone.

For rheumatism and for cramps in the abdomen, I

make use of hay-flowers, as also for complaints of the bladder, and in the first stages of dropsy.

4. Special Vapour Applications on Isolated Spots, such as on the eyes, ears, mouth, fingers, are useful in many cases. A few examples will explain this:—

A venomous insect stings us in the hand; straightway the place swells up, and the inflammation threatens to spread. In conjunction with compresses, a vapour application to the affected spot will bring help and relief.

Whenever there is danger of blood-poisoning from a neglected wound or other cause, a vapour application speedily applied will often arrest the evil.

Sometimes we are attacked with violent cramp at some particular spot of the hand or foot, which may be instantaneously relieved by a vapour application.

Or else you have been bitten by a suspicious-looking dog. Before you have had time to procure a doctor it will be wise to apply vapour to the wound.

Hay-flower infusion is the one I most frequently make use of for outward applications.

For the eyes, an infusion of fennel powder, or else eyebright or milfoil, is serviceable.

For the ears, nettle or milfoil.

For gathering in the throat, decoction of milfoil, ribwort, or nettle.

The duration of these applications is from ten to twenty minutes. All such vapour applications as are made use of for the internal organs, or for eyes and ears, must be employed with caution, and never too hot.

(D) AFFUSIONS.

1. THE KNEE AFFUSION.

The legs being bared to the knee, and the trousers rolled back as far as possible, the patient, seated on a chair, puts his feet into the tub or foot-pail (fig. 11). The affusion is performed by means of a small watering-can from which the rose has been removed, and is light enough to be easily managed with one hand. The contents of the first watering-can, which must be poured faster and stronger than the succeeding ones, moisten both feet from the toes to above the knee. The following cans, which are held alternately high and low, must be directed in such manner as to administer gentle gushes to particular spots; especially the knee-pans and the calves must be watered until the water flows down equally over both feet. The contents of the last watering-can are not poured through the spout, but simply emptied over the feet by way of ablution.

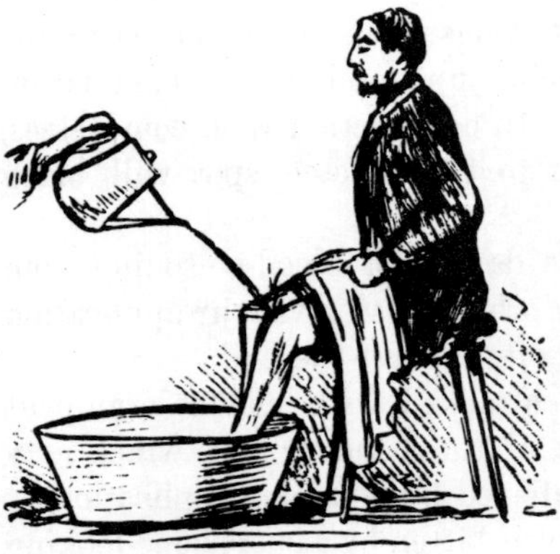

Fig. 11.

For a knee affusion, from two to ten watering-cans full of water may be employed.

Invalids and weak persons can seldom stand the shock of the first affusion,,and to no beginner is the sensation a pleasant one. I have seen strong men, who beforehand had treated the idea with derision, turn pale and tremble like aspen - leaves in vain endeavour to disguise the pain occasioned by the cold-water gush. This potent effect speaks volumes in favour of its invigorating and bracing effects.

Convalescents, and, in general, all such persons as suffer from weakness and poverty of blood, should never attempt more than two to three watering-cans at a time. Novices should begin with two, and then day by day increase the number by two cans more, until they have reached the number of ten. By the eighth watering-can, all sense of pain or discomfort will have disappeared.

The knee affusion is invariably employed in conjunction with the upper affusion, whose description here follows.

2. The Upper Affusion.

The patient strips to the waist, and in order to hinder the water from moistening his under garments, he will do well to protect himself with a towel or sheet wound about the body. The tub or basin which is to receive the down-pouring water is placed on a stool or low chair. The patient leans both hands on the floor of the tub in such manner that the body assumes a horizontal position, and that the water in descending may flow over the body into the vessel (fig. 12).

The contents of the first can, starting from the right arm and right shoulder, descend alongside of the spine to the right, ascending again to the left as far as the shoulder and arm. This first affusion serves to moisten the whole line of action. The contents of the second and of the third are intended to come in contact with the whole network of nerves which extend to both sides of the spine, and, like the first affusion, they must invariably terminate at the left shoulder. The

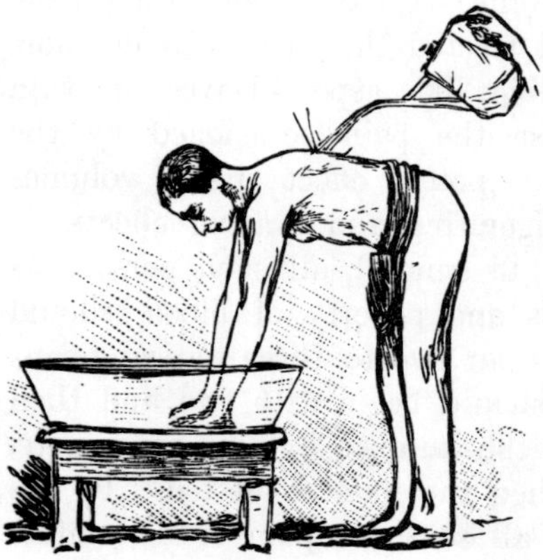

Fig. 12.

whole line must be affused three or four times, as equally as possible, so that the water pours down over the chest into the basin. Let the head be spared, especially if the patient have long hair; the neck, on the contrary, to be well affused. With nervous persons great care must be taken not to affuse the spine itself for long or with too great violence, as the contact of water sometimes causes a pain like that of a sharp stab.

The more rapidly and equally this affusion is performed, the easier it will be to endure, and the faster will warmth be restored to the system.

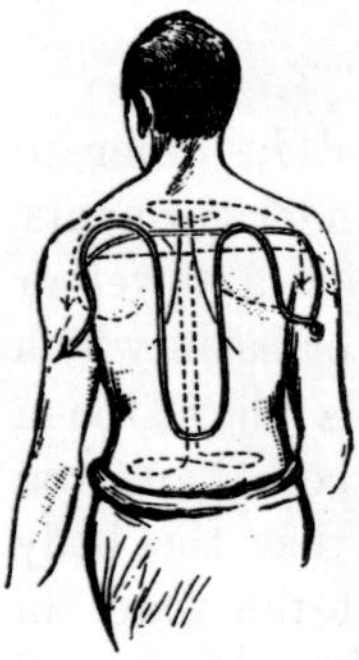

Fig. 13.

With corpulent persons and those who are inclined

to stoutness, reaction is sometimes slow. In such cases I frequently assist the process by rubbing the back gently with the hand after the first affusion: this accelerates the circulation and restores activity to the epidermis.

For the weak, the contents of one watering-can will

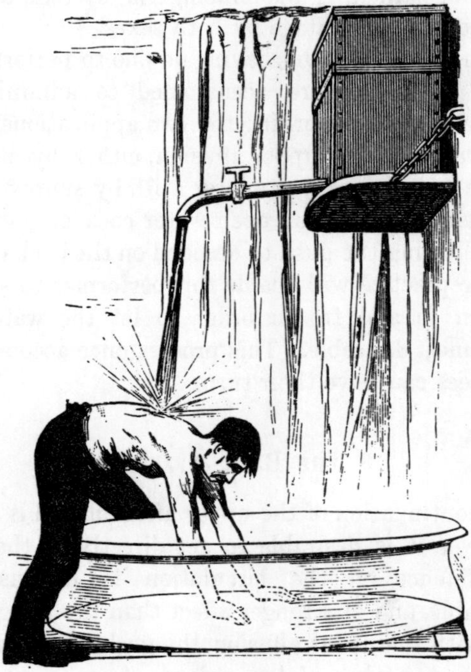

Fig. 14.

be sufficient. For novices one or two, adepts may indulge in from two to three, and the very strong and healthy from five to six watering-cans.

After the affusion let the chest be rapidly washed

over and the clothes resumed without drying the body, whereupon active exercise or work till heat is restored.

The upper affusion must invariably succeed the head vapour bath, but is oftenest used in combination with the knee affusion.

Both affusions take a pre-eminent place among the means of hardening and bracing the system, and may be used with advantage by both sexes.

I know persons who, having no one to perform these offices for them, are accustomed to administer to themselves every morning the two applications. They first undertake the upper affusion, either by means of a little watering-can, or better still, by simply placing themselves beneath an open water cock or pump, and then allowing the gush to descend on the back (fig. 14). A little practice will enable the performer to shift his position to and fro in order to let the water play where most desirable. This process once accomplished the knees can have their turn.

3. The Back Affusion

is the continuation of the upper affusion, and is applied whenever it is desirable to act directly on the spine. Its influence on the circulation is likewise very favourable, and of stronger effect than the foregoing.

As with the upper affusion, the gush here is applied, stronger or weaker, higher or lower, from one shoulder-blade to the other, most particularly, however, on the spine itself, from the cervical vertebræ to the rump-bone or coccyx.

Rapid lavation of chest and under body, as of arms and legs, must always conclude the back affusion.

The simplest method is undoubtedly for the patient to seat himself above a tub or bath in the manner here indicated (fig. 15).

4. The Lower Affusion

is the continuation of the knee affusion, and is so applied, that besides calves and knees, the thighs likewise are to be subjected to the treatment. Its effects are the same as those of the knee affusion, in a more

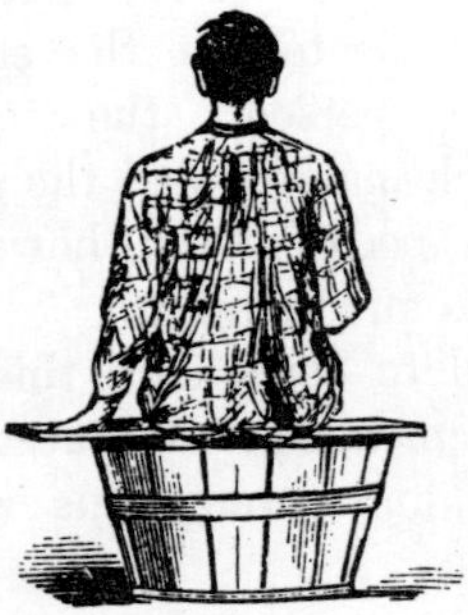

Fig. 15.

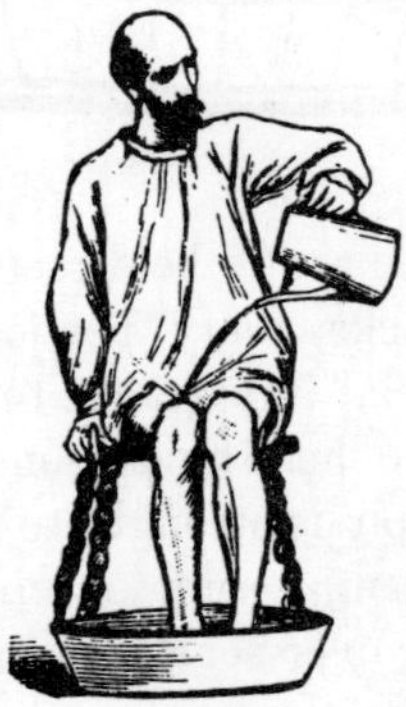

Fig. 16.

potent degree. The lower affusion must invariably succeed the vapour foot-bath, unless preference be given to a semi-bath or to kneeling in water.

This form of affusion is one which any one can apply to himself unassisted (fig. 16).

5. The Complete Affusion

extends to the whole body, as is sufficiently indicated by the title, from the throat to the point of the toes.

It is administered in the following fashion:—

The patient, attired in bathing trousers or shirt, sits in a bath or tub on a narrow board placed across it (fig. 17). The affusions are applied alternately to the chest and the back with the contents of about four watering-cans. The office of the first can is to wet the entire person, the other three are to be directed in such manner that the gush attacks every portion of the body, giving, however, special importance to the spine and stomach.

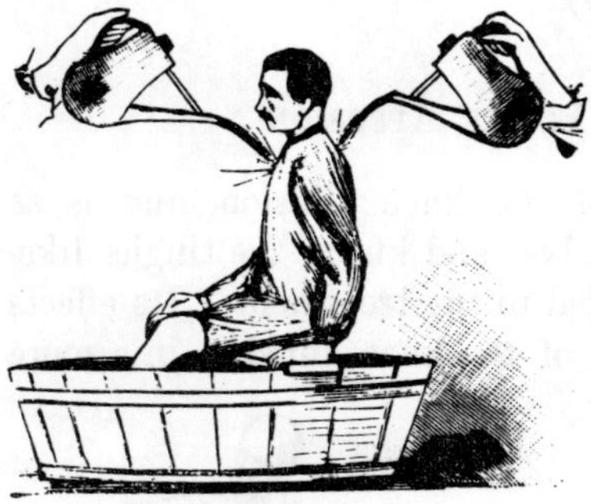

Fig. 17.

To healthy persons inclined to corpulence this affusion is strongly to be recommended. It braces the system, promotes circulation, and strengthens weak and over-sensitive individuals.

For the weak and sickly the water may be tempered to about 66° to 73° F.

One last observation before concluding the chapter on affusions. I am directly opposed to the ultra-violent douches employed in some establishments, not seeing what advantage is to be reaped from such excessive measures. For cleansing the body why should a fire-engine be required? Healthy persons do not require it, and still less the sick.

(*E*) LAVATIONS.

These are divided into whole and partial lavations.

The principal point to be observed with regard to these is, that the water should be applied uniformly and as much as possible equally over the surface of the body or member to be treated. Drying and rubbing are alike prohibited, as in the foregoing applications, and when in describing some particular process I make use of the term "a vigorous lavation," this expression is to be taken as signifying rapidity, not violence of action.

1. Complete Lavation.

(*a*) *Complete Lavation for the Healthy.*

The complete lavation is a rapid ablution applied to the entire body.

The simplest manner of performing it is to dip a coarse linen towel in water, and to begin operations on chest and lower body, proceeding to the back, which each one must approach in the manner he finds most convenient. Arms and legs come last on the programme.

Care should be taken not to perform this operation in a cold or draughty spot, and the general oft-repeated rule of quickly dressing and taking exercise after the application holds likewise good here.

The whole process should not occupy above two minutes.

The early morning is the most favourable time for this lavation. It should be undertaken straight away from the warm bed on rising, and, if possible, be succeeded by a walk in the fresh morning air. Those who have tried it cannot fail to recognise its bracing and invigorating effect.

It is not every one who can with impunity indulge in a cold lavation at night, for with many it has the effect of unduly exciting the nervous system. Those, however, who are able to stand it, will probably find bedtime the most convenient for the process.

Persons suffering from sleeplessness have frequently been relieved by this means.

(b) *Complete Lavation for Invalids.*

The principal point to be observed with regard to the washing of sick people is, that no portion of the body, not even the foot-soles, should remain untouched by the water, which must be rapidly and equally applied over the whole surface.

The patient sits up in bed, or is supported, while back and shoulders are quickly sponged over. Having resumed a horizontal position, chest and body are next attacked, then the arms, and lastly the legs. From three to four minutes at the outside will suffice for the whole operation, which affords speedy and inexpressible relief. Should, however, this complete lavation be too lengthy and fatiguing for very sick persons it may be divided into two or even three partial lavations. Thus chest, body, and arms may be washed in the morning, the back and legs in the afternoon.

The individual application of these lavations is indicated under the chapter of diseases. Let me only here observe that these complete ablutions are of paramount importance in all cases of high fever, more particularly typhus and smallpox.

For the weakly I often prescribe an admixture of vinegar and water, which tends to open and strengthen the pores, and more perfectly to cleanse the body.

2. The Partial Lavation,

as indicated by its name, is applied to one portion merely of the body, and is performed with a coarse linen towel dipped in water. All previous remarks concerning the complete lavation apply equally to the partial lavation.

(*F*) SWATHINGS.

The first of these is termed

1. The Head-swathing.

It can be applied in twofold fashion:—

The whole head, face, and hair included, are washed over so that the water penetrates everywhere, without, however, causing the hair to drip with moisture.

Over the whole head then tie a dry linen cloth, in such manner that it adheres closely and excludes the outer air, leaving only the eyes and half the forehead visible.

Half an hour will usually suffice completely to dry the hair.

The washing and swathing may be repeated as often as three to four times. After the last swathing, the head and neck should be once more quickly washed over.

A still more effective manner of performing this operation, in cases where it is desirable to promote secretion of unhealthy matter, is to wrap a light flannel or woollen shawl above the linen cloth. Likewise, if the head be very hot, it will be advantageous to moisten the linen cloth.

Rheumatic headaches, scurf, and various dry eruptions are readily cured by this swathing.

2. The Throat-swathing.

The milder form of throat-swathing consists in sponging over the whole throat and neck, and then enveloping it in a long narrow linen strip which must be wound three to four times round the neck.

A second and more effective mode is to dip a soft linen towel in water and wind it round the neck; over this a dry towel, and both together to be enveloped in a strip of flannel or a woollen comforter.

My whole experience leads me to reject the over-prolonged application of such swathings and compresses, which mostly defeat their own end by intensifying the heat and disturbing the circulation instead of relieving it.

An hour and a half is the utmost stretch I ever prescribe for the application of a swathing, which must always be renewed at intervals of from twenty minutes to half an hour.

For inflammation of the throat, difficulty in swallowing, &c., this swathing is employed, mostly, however, in conjunction with some other water application, as complete lavation or wet socks.

3. The Shawl.

The shawl is a special form of application for the chest and upper back. It consists in a piece of coarse linen about a yard and a half square (fig. 18), which,

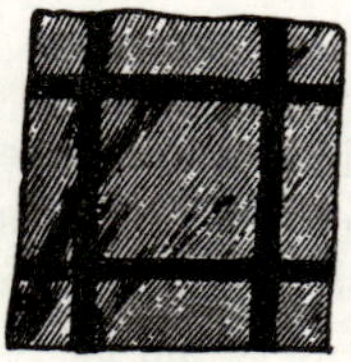

Fig. 18.

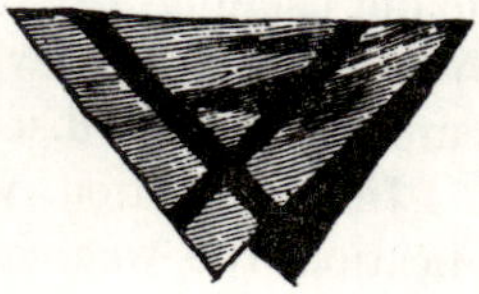

Fig. 19.

dipped in cold water and well wrung out, is folded together to form a triangle (fig. 19), and applied to the patient in guise of a shawl or fichu (figs. 20, 21). A second dry linen cloth, or better still, a flannel or

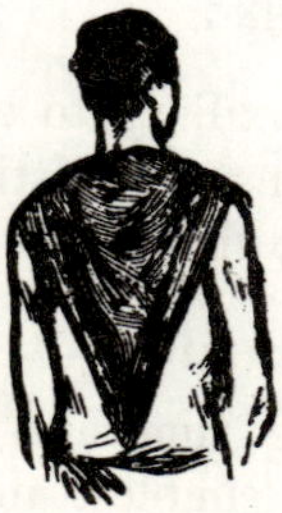

Fig. 20.

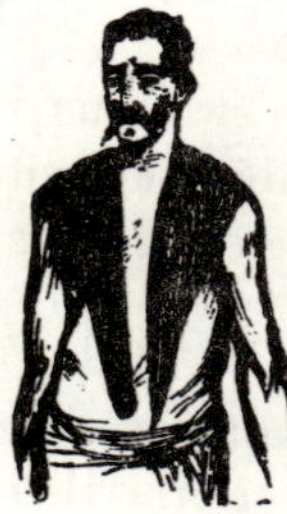

Fig. 21.

woollen shawl, is secured above this in order to exclude the air.

An agreeable sense of warmth will soon be felt by the patient.

The application of the shawl lasts from half an hour to an hour and a half, and may in some special cases be extended to two hours. It should be renewed every half-hour, or whenever the swathing is hot.

For congestions, feverish catarrhs, and in the first stages of inflammation in the head, for gathering in the throat and windpipe obstructions, the shawl will be found useful.

With it I have achieved the most noteworthy results in cures of mental diseases, especially in the weaker sex. In conjunction with a second equally simple application the wet shawl sufficed to withdraw all superfluous blood from the head vessels and to relieve the brain.

This second application just mentioned consisted usually in wet socks or foot-swathings, or else in warm foot-baths with salt and ashes.

4. The Foot-swathing.

This swathing is an important auxiliary, to be used in combination with other applications. We distinguish between two sorts of foot-swathing, viz.—

(a) *The Simple Foot-swathing.*

Country people who have little time and means will perform this operation in the simplest and least troublesome manner by putting on at night a pair of wet socks, and over these again a pair of dry woollen socks or stockings.

Those who object to this proceeding may swaddle their feet in wet linen, above it dry flannel or woollen swathings.

The water in which socks or linen are dipped may be mixed with vinegar, and the application, which should invariably be taken in bed, may last from one to two hours.

Should great heat result from this operation, then the swathing should be renewed at suitable intervals.

In all cases where it is desirable to draw unhealthy secretions from the feet, to reduce inflammation and draw the blood downwards, this swathing will render good service.

Let no one, however, be in danger of confusing the effects of this application with those of the foot-bath, which are of an essentially different nature. The foot-bath is more rapid and transitory in its effects; it serves to draw down the blood from the head, but is powerless to cleanse or secrete unhealthy matter from the body.

Country people returning home at night after a hard day's labour will do well to sleep in wet socks (not forgetting of course to cover these by a pair of dry ones). The wet socks will promote sleep and restore freshness and elasticity to the wearied nerves and muscles. Should you chance, however, to wake up during the night, the soeks must be instantly removed; if not, they should be taken off the first thing in the morning.

The foot-swathing may also be used with advantage by those who suffer from cold feet. For profuse perspiration of the feet it is likewise to be recommended, but only in conjunction with the vapour foot-bath.

(*b*) *Swathing above the knee* is of stronger effect than the preceding, and is applied in the same fashion, with the difference that the wrapping is prolonged to above the knee.

For the length of this application and all other instructions regarding it, the remarks regarding simple foot-swathing hold good.

For withdrawing the heat from the upper body in cases of great fatigue, and removing unhealthy winds and gases, I can warmly recommend this swathing.

5. The Lower Swathing

is thus called because it is chiefly employed for diseases of the legs and lower body. . It begins under the arms, and reaches till over the toes. The upper chest, shoulders, and arms remaining free, must be carefully covered over to secure the patient from cold.

The lower swathing is prepared in the following manner:—

A large thick woollen blanket is spread over the mattress; above it the wet sheet well wrung out, and which must be large enough to envelop the body in

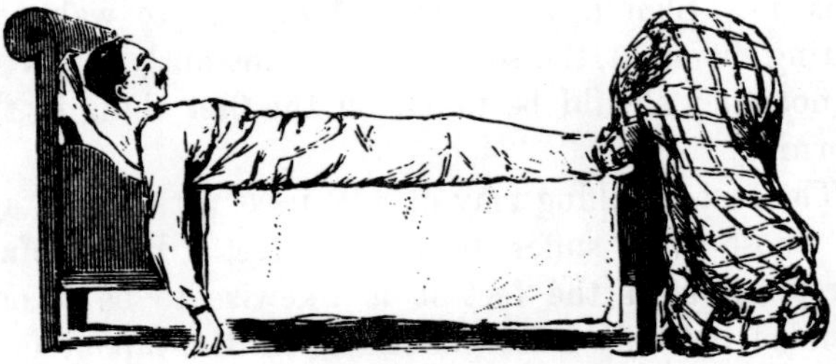

Fig. 22.

two to three fold fashion. The patient lies down on the spread-out sheet, which is then closely folded over him to the right and left until every portion of the lower body comes in contact with the wet linen (fig. 22).

The blanket is then wrapped over so as to form a complete protection against the outer air. The whole person is then covered with a feather quilt, in addition to which an extra rug or blanket may be placed over the feet.

The duration of this application is from one to two hours. Persons who have an insurmountable dislike to cold water, as well as the aged and weak, may employ lukewarm water for this purpose.

Country people and peasants often simplify the process by taking an old sack, which, having dipped in water and well wrung out, they draw on over the whole person up to the arm-pits. Thus attired they lie down and are covered up with blankets or feather quilts.

The action of this swathing, which is always made use of in conjunction with other applications, is threefold: it promotes heat, dissolves and secretes the germs of unhealthy matter contained in the system. For tumours on the legs, rheumatic and gouty affections, flatulency, cramps, &c., it is a valuable auxiliary.

Instead of simple cold or warm water I often make use of an infusion of hay-flowers, sour hay, oat-straw, or pine-needles. The sour hay is a substitute for hay-flowers, and both are efficient in cases of difficult urination; also, in a minor degree, they have a favourable influence on gravel and stone complaints.

The infusion of oat-straw has done good service in cases of gout, gravel, and stone.

The pine-tree infusion is chiefly for the weakly; it is useful for flatulency and cramps of the abdomen.

6. The Short Swathing

is the one most universally employed, and the most independent of all cold-water applications, inasmuch as it depends upon the assistance of no other. Being easily applied and of excellent effect, it well deserves to be a general favourite.

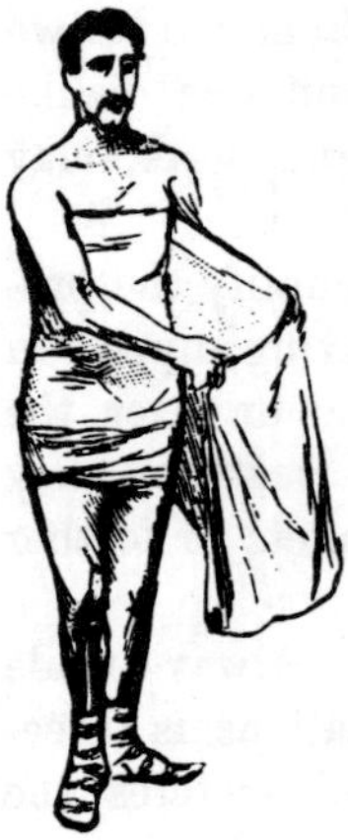

Fig. 23.

A coarse linen sheet folded together four to six fold is dipped in water and wound closely round the body from the armpits to the centre of the thighs (fig. 23); above it a piece of flannel or woollen stuff, and the patient is covered up in bed as in the foregoing applications.

For the aged and weak, warm water may be employed.

An old sack folded together to the requisite width may be made to serve the purpose of poor country people.

If healthy people would but make use of this short swathing once a-week, or even once a-fortnight, how many illnesses might not thereby be averted! It acts favourably on liver and kidneys, and brings relie in heart, stomach, and dropsical complaints, by dispelling superfluous gases.

Whenever I am in doubt as to the nature of a complaint and wish to ascertain the exact seat of the evil, I always find the short swathing to be my best and truest counsellor.

Patients who suffer from weakness of the abdomen

should rub their body, either before or after the application, with oil of camphor, or lard.

For cramps I sometimes make use of a cloth dipped in pure vinegar and placed single-fold against the body under the wet wrapper.

7. The Wet Shirt.

I have selected this application as being sufficiently self-evident to be grasped by the meanest intelligence.

A common linen shirt is dipped in water, well wrung out, and put on by the patient, who goes to bed, having wrapped himself in a thick woollen blanket and sufficiently covered himself with rugs or quilts.

The wet shirt may be kept on from one to two hours. It acts like a very mild form of blister, and has the effect of opening the pores, relieving cramps and congestion, and soothing the nervous system. I have employed it with great effect in mental diseases, and on children attacked with St Vitus's dance. In many skin-diseases it is eminently valuable; and in cases of scarlet fever, measles, &c., when it is an object to promote the eruption and bring it to the surface, I make use of a shirt dipped in salt water or an admixture of vinegar.

8. The Spanish Mantle.

This pompous appellation is not of my invention, but, being in common use, it may as well serve my purpose here.

The Spanish mantle, likewise called "large swathing," is a sort of long cloak with sleeves made of coarse linen, cut very wide and long, and open up the front. Perhaps it would be more correct to designate it as a coarse linen dressing-gown (fig. 24). This cloak, dipped in water,—which can be warm or cold according to the particular case,—is put on by the patient, who wraps it tightly about him and goes to bed as previously described (fig. 25).

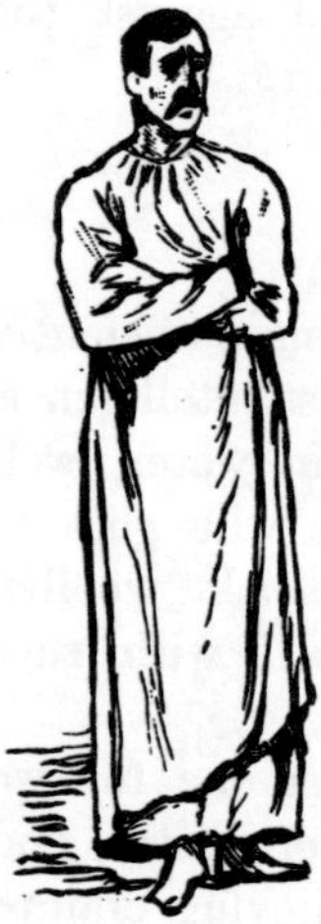

Fig. 24.

The duration of this application is from one to two hours, and must be regulated by the patient's strength—more particularly, however, by his size and weight. For a thin gaunt peasant one hour will suffice; a burgomaster or an alderman may unhesitatingly indulge in two hours.

Whoever wishes to ascertain how potent are the effects of the Spanish mantle need only examine the

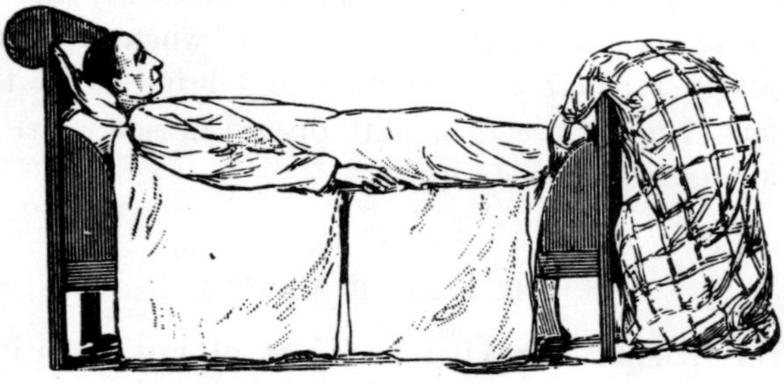

Fig. 25.

water in which the cloak has been rinsed out after the application. The water will be found to be dull and discoloured; and I have known cases where the linen cloak itself was dyed throughout of a yellow hue, which could only be removed by bleaching.

I specially make use of the Spanish mantle in cases of general catarrh (where it extends over the whole system), for slime-fever, gout, smallpox, typhus, and as a preventive against apoplexy. In Part III. of this work we shall frequently meet the Spanish mantle.

Dipped in an infusion of hay-flowers, oat-straw, or pine-needles, it is of excellent effect in various diseases, such as gravel, stone, &c., according to the individual effects of each of these plants.

(*G*) WATER-DRINKING.

This paragraph may be a brief one. I warn everybody against the two extremes—that of drinking too much and of not drinking at all. Some years ago it was the fashion to imbibe large quantities of water by way of cure—a daily allowance of four, six, eight, and even ten pints being of common practice; and even now there are many who entertain an undefined notion that much water-drinking must be conducive to health.

Those of the second category hold a diametrically opposite opinion, and pass days, weeks, and even months without anything in the shape of fluid crossing their lips.

Are not both these proceedings equally senseless?

Before the clock strikes it gives us warning, and does not the greatest of all mechanicians, the Creator, do the same by all His creatures? He gives us hunger as a sign that it is time to eat, and thirst to tell us when we should drink. The human system, that living clock of exquisitely accurate construction, would ever move and strike with unfailing punctuality were it not for the blindness of mankind, which soils the works, and obstructs their rotation by dust and dirt.

Wild and tame animals eat and drink whenever they experience thirst or hunger, and desist when they are satisfied; and a rational unvitiated human being will act in like manner.

Drink, therefore, whenever thou art thirsty, and never drink much at a time!

I know persons who hardly ever drink from week's end to week's end; others to whom a glass of water at breakfast is sufficient for the whole day. This may easily be explained by the fact that in every dish of which we partake a certain amount of liquid is contained. Except during the great heat in midsummer, or a feverish state of the system, thirst is an element foreign to many people; and it always is to me a mystery wherefore so many persons, without the slightest necessity, choose to flood their poor stomachs with whole deluges of liquid! Such a course cannot fail to bring its revenge in time.

At this place I wish to say a few words about drinking during meals. This applies to those in the more civilised walks of life, for with peasants and country people drinking at table is not a general habit.

Our food, as we chew it in the mouth, should be penetrated throughout with the saliva, which has specially been given to us for the purpose of assisting digestion.

If, therefore, we dilute this valuable sap with another fluid, such as water, beer, or wine, we necessarily weaken its effects.

When and how should we therefore drink?

Let him drink who is thirsty before meals, for the thirst is then a sure indication of scanty or thick saliva, which requires to be diluted and renewed.

During meals we should as much as possible, refrain from drinking, in order that everything we eat may be thoroughly amalgamated with the pure saliva.

When a certain time has elapsed after a meal, digestion again demands a renewal of the stomach saps. In other words, if in one, two, or three hours after eating we feel thirsty, it is permissible to drink in moderation.

Drink as often as thou art thirsty, and never drink to excess!

The peasants do not care for violent sudden showers of rain, for they declare that such do more harm than good, and render the land unfruitful. Those heavy morning mists, on the contrary, which wet the hat till it drips with moisture, are the peasants' best friends, for they promote fertility.

It has lately become the fashion to praise the effects of warm water imbibed at the temperature of 100° to 111° F. for certain chronic diseases. I have myself employed this remedy in former years, and not without success. Let honour be given to whomsoever honour is due, and far be it from me to condemn those who prefer hot water to the pure cold element.

My experience, however, is all in favour of cold water, which I consider to be capable of achieving equal, if not superior, results to those obtainable with warm. This question is entirely one of individual taste; let each person, therefore, select that which he finds most congenial.

PART II.

PHARMACY

"*Benedicite universa germinantia in terra Domino!*"

INTRODUCTORY REMARKS.

I AM a sworn enemy of all secret remedies and patent medicines, whose composition and ingredients are enveloped in mystery.

This reproach cannot be addressed to me. I willingly throw open the drawers of my pharmacy and invite every one to analyse their contents. No expensive stock-in-trade will be found here, for most of my medicines, infusions, extracts, oils, and powders are drawn from simple weeds and herbs, well known and much prized by our ancestors, but mostly now forgotten and despised. These may be found in almost every field and garden, on the common, and by the wayside; and as this little work is chiefly written for the poor, the greatest merit of my remedies lies in their very cheapness and vulgarity.

It is for the sake of the poor that I have devoted long years to this study, seeking out and renewing acquaintance with each obscure and insignificant herb, with a view to raising it anew to well-deserved honour and consideration. I have examined and analysed, dried and dissected, boiled and tasted each over and over again. There is no herb, no powder, whose effects have not been previously tried on myself before giving it to the world.

I was long in doubt as to whether or not I should publish the result of these botanical experiments as appendix to my cold-water cure, being, as I am, fully persuaded that cold water alone is sufficient to cure all complaints. There are, however, many persons who shrink from the prospect of a prolonged cold-water cure, and for these this portion of the book is written. By help of the remedies here indicated the water applications may be curtailed and simplified.

To those plants whose action appeared to me doubtful, such as marsh-mallow or liquorice, I have accorded little attention. Poisonous plants have been completely omitted from my pharmacy.

How good is God towards us! my heart impels me to exclaim here. Not only that which we require for sustaining life, our daily bread, does He cause to grow for us. In unerring wisdom He has created everything in perfect measure and harmony, and His paternal love makes countless little herbs spring up from the earth in order to bring solace and consolation to suffering mankind.

How good is God! If only we had sense to recognise it! Let us pursue attentively the little plants to which the Creator has given scent, as a tiny perfume-flask, by which to proclaim their qualities and attract our attention; and as we pluck them, let us render thanks to our Father in heaven, who provides so bountifully for His children.

Our household pharmacy should contain four principal partitions, and several smaller side partitions.

The four principal partitions consist of—

Tinctures or extracts.
Tea-infusions.
Powders.
Oils.

Into the side partitions, properly sorted and arranged, comes everything else which cannot be classified under the foregoing four heads. Also linen rags and cotton wool for dressing wounds should find here a place.

The tinctures and oils must be kept in glasses or bottles; teas and powders in close paper bags, or, better still, in wooden boxes. If these are ordered new for this purpose, they should be oval-shaped, and of different sizes. If they are all made of a uniform pattern, this will give the household pharmacy a business-like, neat appearance, and it will be a pleasure to look at them ranged upon the shelves like a well-disciplined army of soldiers.[1] Everything to be kept in a dry, cool, and easily accessible place.

The contents of each glass bottle, bag, or box should be distinctly marked on a label affixed to it, and it will save both time and trouble if these are arranged alphabetically.

Great order, method, and cleanliness are the principal conditions for organising and keeping up this household pharmacy. It should be presided over by the mother of the family, or else by her most tidy and industrious son or daughter. Well governed and administered, this little pharmacy will be a source of blessing and consolation to the whole household; and

[1] **Old toy-boxes may, however, very well serve the purpose.—Translator's note.**

its faithful dispenser may joyfully remember the words of our blessed Saviour, "Inasmuch as ye have done it unto one of the least of these my brethren, ye have done it unto me" (Matt. xxv. 40).

At the end of this part I have given a list of the contents of the pharmacy, from which I have banished everything of a superfluous nature.

A word more here as to the preparation of tinctures, teas, powders, and oils.

Tinctures or Extracts.

The healing virtues of a plant, its inward sap, may be extracted in various ways. The best and most potent extraction may be obtained as follows:—

Among the herbs, berries, or flowers from which the medicine is to be made, seek out the most perfect specimens, ripe and undecayed; these are to be well dried in the open air upon a wooden board or tray —placed, however, *in the shade*, never in the sun.

When everything is well dried, cut up or pull asunder those that require to be diminished in size, and place everything in a clean, easily corked glass bottle. Over this pour pure corn-brandy or some other kind of unadulterated spirit. Well close the bottle and place for a time in a moderately warm spot. The longer the extract is kept, the stronger it will be, and I often make use of a tincture after it has stood a year undisturbed. In case of necessity, however, it may be used after a few days.

The tinctures are to be administered in drops; sometimes (when expressly indicated) in tea- or even tablespoonfuls.

The qualities of all berries, herbs, and flowers which are employed as tinctures may also be expressed in wine. This wine, however, is not intended to be kept any length of time, but is mostly employed for immediate use.

TEAS.

In dry weather, when you are coming back from the fields, or when going out to view the state of the crops, turn aside occasionally from your path to pluck here and there one of the healing herbs. Give the preference to those that grow on dry soil—best of all, on sunny hillsides; and those flowers and berries which are most perfectly expanded and developed, will bring you the best fruits in time of sickness. Many of the plants and herbs will be found growing in your own kitchen-garden, near the house or farm buildings. Teach your ten-year-old little girl or boy how to seek for the plants; this will give them pleasure and save your own time.

The plants should every year be renewed—that is to say, a new stock gathered in and the old ones thrown away.

Each housewife knows how to prepare tea: for one cupful, she takes of the dried herbs as flowers as much as she can grasp in three fingers, pours over it boiling water, and lets it boil up once or twice. After straining, it will then be ready for use.

Made in this fashion, the tea will have the most delicate pleasing taste, but it will not be of the strongest kind.

My method of making it is different. I let it boil for long, until every particle of strength is extracted from the plant, in order that none of its healing virtues may be wasted.

How and when these teas are to be administered, I have indicated at the proper place.

Powders.

A powder is obtained by scraping or pounding in a mortar the dry roots, leaves, berries, or seeds.

Many sick people prefer to take medicine in this shape to swallowing cupfuls of fluid. It may be strewn over their food or mixed with their drink in such fashion that they never suspect its presence.

The glasses or boxes where these powders are kept should be air-tight.

Oils.

The different oils appertaining to the pharmacy can be bought ready-made of the apothecary in every country town or village.

As with the other medicines, the oil-bottles should be kept clean and in good order.

MEDICAMENTS.

ALMOND-OIL.

THE oil of sweet almonds should rank first among the oils contained in the household pharmacy.

It is useful in cases of conglutination of the stomach and windpipe, dissolving the slime and restoring appetite.

It cools inflammation, especially the redoubtable inflammation of the lungs. Patients attacked with this illness should daily take three to four teaspoonfuls of the oil internally.

For earache, cramp, or wind in the ear, and other like complaints, six to eight drops may be poured into the suffering ear, which must then be carefully closed with cotton wool.

Those who suffer from deafness in consequence of catching cold, or from a rheumatic affection, should employ seven to eight drops daily on each ear in alternation. After continuing this practice for several days, the ear should be washed out with lukewarm water, or, better still, syringed by a proficient hand.

Boils which are attended by much heat may be gently rubbed over with almond-oil.

It is also a good thing with which to rub the skin when you are "saddle-sick," or to apply to any part of the body which is chafed or sore.

In default of almond-oil, olive-oil may be employed.

Aloe.

This powder (which can be bought at the apothecary's) is of good effect for both inward and outward use. One to two pinches of aloe-powder mixed with a teaspoonful of honey will serve to cleanse the stomach without producing irritation.

Combined with other herbs, and infused as tea, it is of yet greater effect. The mixture is usually as follows: One pinch of aloe, sufficient elder-flowers for two cups of tea, two pinches of fenugreek, a teaspoonful of fennel. The two cups of tea are to be taken in the course of two days. Their action in promoting stools does not take place till from twelve to thirty hours later.

Outwardly applied it is good for weak, red, and suppurated eyes. A good pinch of aloe infused in boiling water will make an excellent eye-water, which can be used from three to four times daily. It may also be applied to old wounds, proud flesh, and deep scars which have suppurated, by dipping a linen in this water and placing it on the affected part.

Aloe (*Aloe vulgaris*).

This plant, which many people keep in their rooms by way of ornament, has got thick long leaves which are covered with prickly spikes. If every one knew the value of these leaves, no home would be without at least one such plant.

A leaf of the aloe boiled in water will produce a medicine a cupful of which will cleanse stomach and bowels. Reduced to powder, two pinches daily will act beneficially in liver complaints and jaundice.

A spoonful of honey boiled with an aloe-leaf in a pint of water will, if taken in small doses, remove internal heat, and heal sore gums, especially if these be the result of whooping-cough.

Mixed with wormwood, it serves to secrete watery saps which might otherwise have turned to dropsy.

Alum.

Alum is of corrosive action, and is suitable for indolent tumours and wounds. I have seen cases when an early stage of cancer was averted by means of alum.

The application is as follows:—

The alum is either reduced to powder and then sprinkled over the wound, or else dissolved in water: it is applied to the affected part by means of linen rags dipped in the solution.

A weak solution of alum-water is good for sore and diseased gums. It may likewise be used for gargling.

Angelica (*Angelica silvestris*, L.)

Upon damp meadows and in the woods we find a plant which grows to the height of from 20 to 40 inches. It has a hollow stem, out of which the boys like to make pipes. The name of this plant is Angelica. Its healing powers on the human system are unfortunately too little known. If any one has partaken of poisonous or unwholesome food, a tea made of the roots, seeds, and leaves of this plant will be found an excellent remedy, as it tends to remove and secrete the unhealthy matter.

How often we feel a sensation of cold in the stomach! A cup of tea made of these roots will quickly restore the internal warmth. It is best to imbibe such a cupful in three portions, to be taken morning, noon, and night.

Flatulency and unwholesome gases in stomach and bowels are readily cured by a cup of this tea, especially if the tea be infused with a mixture of wine-and-water. For congestion in lungs, windpipe, and chest, and for burning pains in the stomach, it is likewise very serviceable.

The dried roots, leaves, and seeds may be reduced to powder, and thus employed instead of the tea.

ANISEED (*Pimpinella anisum*, L.)

Aniseed, like fennel, may be warmly recómmended. Its action upon unwholesome gases and flatulency is even greater than that of fennel. Oftenest these two remedies are employed combined together.

Oil of aniseed and of fennel may be bought in every apothecary's. For the afore-named complaints four to seven drops on sugar once or twice daily will suffice.

ARNICA (*Arnica montana*, L.)

Tincture of arnica is so well known for its healing and strengthening effects upon wounds, sprains, &c., as hardly to require any commentary.

It is not expensive to buy, but any one can prepare it for himself. The blossoms, collected at the end of June or beginning of July, are placed in air-tight bottles into which corn-brandy or spirits are poured. In three days the tincture will be ready for use.

Ashes.

Wood-ashes are always employed for medical purposes: those of lime-wood being the best and finest. The fresher they are, the more effective they will be; those just withdrawn from the hearth will be best of all.

After illnesses in which the digestive organs have suffered we derive much benefit from ashes. This may sound peculiar, but is true nevertheless. Powdered ashes are easiest taken mixed in milk with a little sugar; and the daily portion, which should not exceed one table-spoonful, may be taken all at once, or divided into two doses.

Consumptive patients may daily drink two pints of milk, each pint containing a spoonful of ground ashes.

It may likewise be powdered over old suppurated sores and wounds, as it will assist the healing process.

Bilberry (*Vaccinium myrtillus*).

About the time of St James's feast (25th July), the children love to go to the forest: the bilberries are ripe, a prime delicacy for these young brats. Even grown-up children do not despise these dark-hued berries, and we see them piled up in baskets in the town market-place. Their sight will remind many a student of bygone happy childish days, when he used to pluck bilberries with his little sister, and perchance he will sometimes stop and buy a few coppers' worth of the fruit for the sake of "auld lang syne."

No household should be without a good supply of

dried bilberries throughout the year: they will be found useful in manifold cases.

Good corn-brandy poured over two to three handfuls of bilberries in a bottle, will produce an extract which may be kept for years, and will improve with keeping.

Obstinate diarrhœa may be relieved by a spoonful of bilberry extract, taken in a gill of warm water, and repeated after 8 to 10 hours. It will hardly be necessary to repeat the dose a third time.

Even in cases of severe dysentery, the bilberry extract will be found of good service, used in conjunction with compresses of vinegar and water.

The dose must be regulated according to the nature and violence of the disease; 10 to 30 drops on sugar being the smallest, one tea-spoonful, taken in warm water or wine, the largest, dose.

BONE-DUST (*see* CHALK).

Of this bone-dust I always prepare three sorts—viz.:

(*a*) *Black Powder.*

I take clean bones of a healthy ox, and expose these to the glowing heat until the bones are reduced to ashes. These black ashes must be pounded fine, and a very simple efficacious remedy will be complete.

(*b*) *White Powder.*

I burn the bones until they have assumed the appearance of quick-set lime; pound as above, the result being a powder which has the appearance of pipeclay.

(c) *Grey Powder*

is composed of a mixture of the black and white dust, producing a grey-hued powder.

Those who read my remarks under the heading Chalk, will understand why I attach great importance to bone-dust.

Its effects are most noteworthy after severe illness, when the patient is much weakened. I am often unable to restrain my own astonishment at the wonderful results achieved by it.

Many may fail to understand wherefore I prepare three separate sorts of powder out of the same bone. I do this because each separate preparation is adapted to a different phase of weakness.

To convalescents who suffer from general weakness of the system, and to little children who seem to be dwindling away like stunted treelets, I administer one to two pinches of the black powder daily in water, or mixed in the food.

Patients of whom I note that their machinery works slow and indolently, that their circulation and digestion are out of order, that their bones in especial appear to be in shaken condition like that of a crumbling building, receive the white bone-dust.

The mixture of the two powders is administered to those patients, or convalescents, whose internal organs and vessels are much weakened.

This, dear reader, is the whole secret of the black, white, and grey powders, of whose effects so many patients are able to relate, and which have been so much discussed and disputed over. Believe me, these powders alone might have made me a rich man. But

I detest and despise all secret remedies, which are justly to be regarded as quacksalving swindles. My remedies need not fear the open light of day. Let each one examine for himself and select the best.

Bran.

Instead of throwing this into the pigs'-trough, as so many senseless people are in the habit of doing, they should rather save this noble, nutritious, and wholesome substance for their own weak and suffering children.

Nothing is more welcome to convalescents, weaklings, and children than easily digested food, and the weakest stomach is capable of retaining a decoction of bran, which is, so to say, the very quintessence of the grain itself. Let no one be surprised at this assertion: it is a well-known fact that the rinds of apples and pears possess more strength than the actual fruit.

Take wheat or corn bran and boil it for three-quarters of an hour in water; then press out the bran and strain; mix honey into the decoction, and boil up again for half an hour. Of this drink the patient may take twice daily half a pint. White bread or roll dipped in it will be pleasant to the taste.

For children, and for the aged, I know no better, more wholesome beverage, and those who have tried it will sing its praises.

If we would but strive to become simpler, more rational, more frugal in our habits! God grant that it may be so! for much depends upon it.

CAMOMILE (*Matricaria chamomilla*, L.)

Camomile tea, for colds, catarrhs, especially when these are attended by fever; for stomach-pain, cramps, violent congestion, toothache,—is a well-known and trusty friend in every (German) house. Less familiar to the English public will probably be the little muslin bags filled with dried camomile flowers, which will relieve pain when applied warm on the stomach or abdomen.

CAMPHOR.

The properties of camphor are well known. Its effects are soothing and pain-stilling.

It may be used as spirits of camphor or camphor-oil.

For spirits of camphor, dissolve a piece as large as a hazel nut in half a pint of spirits. It is only for outward application,—to be rubbed on the affected part in cases of bruises, sprains, rheumatic and spasmodical complaints. Many people employ it merely for strengthening some particular limb or part, and they act rightly in so doing.

Camphor-oil is produced by mixing powdered camphor in almond or salad oil. It is excellent for rubbing in, in cases of rheumatism, gout, and pains in the back.

CENTAURY (*Erithrea centaurium*, L.)

Is called in German *Tausendguldenkraut* — literally, the thousand florin herb. How curiously certain herbs have been christened by our ancestors! The reason of this is that they knew their now forgotten worth. Our little flower must have occupied a high social position in the herbal world of those bygone days.

Its taste is bitter, and its mission, employed as tea, is to relieve the stomach of superfluous winds and gases, to restore the digestive saps, and act upon liver and kidneys. It is the best remedy for heartburn. Sufferers from derangement of the circulation may seek counsel and help from the herb.

CHALK (*see* BONE-DUST).

Every one must have seen how, not only foals but other household animals, are fond of swallowing little particles of lime or mortar; and who has not heard of children from whom the schoolroom chalk had to be hidden away, lest they should break up and greedily devour it?

Does not nature give us hereby a hint as to the beneficial action of chalk upon the human system? I myself have made use of chalk in large quantities with quite surprising results.

Chalk contains sulphur, lime, and other ingredients; let us call these at once building materials, which often serve to strengthen and build up anew the marvellous edifice constructed by the greatest of all architects.

To weaklings and children I give daily a pinch of chalk in water, or mixed with the food. Being absolutely tasteless and scentless, powdered chalk is easily swallowed. Let those who suffer from imperfect digestion, and children who in spite of all care do not seem to thrive, give chalk a trial, taken as above.

It is specially efficacious in green sickness. Those affected with this complaint should take not one but two pinches daily, morning and evening. This white powder will soon change the patients' pale faces to a healthy red. More potent in its effects than chalk is bone-dust.

Cloves, Oil of.

Oil of cloves is employed in the same manner as almond or olive oil, and is often mixed with these.

I have found it to be of special use against indolent gases and unhealthy saps in the stomach.

The dose, to be taken on sugar, is from four to six drops, once or twice daily.

Coltsfoot (*Tussilago petasitis* and *farfara*).

Many plants like the coltsfoot seem to have been created but to be trodden under foot, but those who are acquainted with its qualities will hold this plant in high esteem.

Coltsfoot-tea is excellent for clearing and cleansing chest and lungs; for cough and for all those who incline to consumption. Fresh coltsfoot-leaves laid on the chest will draw out heat and fever, and may also be used for open wounds.

They are specially serviceable for open sores on the feet, when the spots are highly inflamed, blue or black in hue. They draw out heat and pain, and expel the unhealthy matter. Also for erysipelas they may be used with advantage.

Coltsfoot-leaves may be dried in the shade, rubbed down to powder, and taken as medicine; the dose is from one to two pinches, taken two or three times daily. This powder, like many others, may be mixed with the patient's food.

Cowslip (*Primula officinalis*, L.)

Only the dark-yellow cowslip is of any value for the household pharmacy. Its mere scent reveals to us that it must be gifted with peculiar virtues. It suffices to chew two or three of these little yellow cups, in order to guess the medicinal qualities here concealed.

Shooting pains in the limbs may readily be cured by a daily cupful of cowslip tea. This cure should be continued for some length of time.

Danewort or Dwarf-Elder (*Sambucus ebulus*, L.)

At the forest edge, especially there where the wood has been cut down, we find a shrub growing to the height of a yard which in spring-time bears large umbelliferous white blossoms, in autumn a rich burden of shining corymbiferous berries. This is the danewort or dwarf-elder bush. Its berries are smaller than those of the household elder, but they are far more numerous, and the plant is hardier than its more civilised brother.

Tea of the danewort root is of special service for expelling the water in dropsy, and in purifying the kidneys. In my own experience several cases of advanced dropsy have been completely arrested and cured by this means.

It is likewise useful for other complaints of the abdomen having their origin in unhealthy saps, which it secretes through the urine.

Danewort tea, prepared with the powder of danewort, is similar in its effects. For one cupful, to be taken in two separate doses on the same day, two pinches of the powder will suffice.

In late autumn the roots should be collected, carefully dried in the open air, and put aside for winter use.

ELDER, BLACK (*Sambucus nigra*, L.)

In the good old times the elder-bush used to stand nearest to the house; now it has mostly been dislodged from this familiar position. No home should be without this faithful guardian, whose leaves, blossoms, berries, and bark all contain valuable properties.

With returning spring, vigorous natures seek to disembarrass themselves of certain saps and matter which during winter have accumulated in the system. Who has not experienced this feeling, which has been termed the spring sickness, often accompanied by eruptions, diarrhœa, colic, and similar complaints?

Those who wish to undertake a slight spring cure, and to secrete unhealthy matter from blood and body, should take from six to eight fresh leaves of the elder-tree, cut these up small after the manner of tobacco, and let the tea boil up for ten minutes. One cupful daily, taken an hour before breakfast during some length of time, will suffice for the cure.

This cure may also be undertaken at any other time of the year, and in default of fresh leaves, dried ones may be used.

People inclined to dropsy should drink elder-root tea. This infusion has the effect of secreting the superfluous water in large quantities.

The berries are often cooked in autumn and made into a sort of frumenty or pap, much prized by our ancestors for its effects in cleansing the blood. My deceased mother used to perform this elder-root cure every year for two to three weeks. It was for this reason that our forefathers always planted some elder-trees in the vicinity of the house.

As nowadays genteel folks wander forth to distant countries to perform the costly grape-cure, so used our parents and grand-parents to consult the adjacent elder-tree, which served them as well and with far less expense and trouble.

Even the birds, before they migrate in autumn, seek out the elder-tree in order to purify their blood and gather strength for the long journey. What a pity it is that men have lost this healthy natural instinct!

Boiled with sugar or honey for winter use, the elder-berries will be found valuable for persons whose occupation forces them to lead a sedentary life. A spoonful of this jam, stirred into a glass of water, will give an excellent cooling and refreshing drink: it cleanses the stomach, promotes water, and acts favourably on the kidneys.

Many country people dry the berries, which can be used as tea or pap. Used in whatever shape, it is always efficacious in cases of violent laxation.

The good services formerly rendered by the elder-tree have been so completely forgotten, that this trusty household benefactor has frequently been exiled or destroyed.

May the good old friend rise again to renewed honour and consideration!

EYEBRIGHT (*Euphrasia officinalis*, L.)

In gratitude, and as a reward for its valuable services, our ancestors bestowed the pretty name of

Augentrost (literally, consolation of the eye) on this little herb. Often, when other means were unavailing, this flower has procured a last consolation to suffering eyes. I have frequently made use of it, and with good results.

When the aftermath is half-grown, about August, you will find this medicinal herb on almost every meadow, where it sometimes sprouts so profusely, to the detriment of the actual crop, as to arouse the peasant's ire.

Both dried and grated leaves are respectively employed for making tea and powder. With the tea, daily wash out the eyes two to three times, or else with it moisten linen rags, which are laid on the eyes overnight, and secured by a bandage. The eye will be purified, cleared, and the vision strengthened.

Experience has taught me to employ the eyebright powder simultaneously as an internal remedy. One pinch daily, administered in water or soup, is the proper dose. We have not yet exhausted the list of the eyebright's virtues. It might well deserve also to be called consolation of the stomach. Eyebright tea is an excellent stomachic: by reason of its innate bitterness, it promotes digestion and improves the stomach saps. Give it a trial, dear reader: this little herb will freely dispense to you likewise its beneficent consolation.

Fennel (*Fœniculum officinale*, L.)

Fennel seeds should never be wanting in the household pharmacy, the complaints which they serve to cure being of common occurrence. By this I mean colic, with all its attendant cramps and spasms. Let the mother quickly boil one table-spoonful of fennel in a cup of milk from five to ten minutes, and give the healing beverage to the patient as hot as can conveniently be swallowed. Its action is good, and mostly very rapid.

Fennel powder, strewed upon, or mixed with the food, expels unhealthy gases from the stomach and other regions. It is made by roasting the seeds in the oven and grinding them in a common coffee-mill.

Fennel oil can be bought of the apothecary.

Fennel employed as eye-water will be familiar to many. It is produced by boiling half a tea-spoonful of fennel powder in water, and washing the eyes thrice daily with the decoction.

Of more potent effect is the fennel vapour eye-bath, which has been already explained.

Aniseed and caraway have much the same effect as fennel. Sometimes all these three kind of seeds are employed together.

Fenugreek (*Trigonella fœnum græcum*, L.)

Powder made of fenugreek seeds gives a valuable tea of cooling effect in fever.

For sore throat attended with much heat it is an excellent gargle. One tea-spoonful of this powder suffices for an average-sized cup of tea, of which a table-spoonful may be taken every hour either as drink or as gargle.

Employed externally, fenugreek is the best remedy I know to use for boils and swellings, with a view to bringing these to a head. Its action is slow and painless, but thorough in its effects. The seeds are boiled down to a sort of pap, as in the case of linseed, and applied as poultice to the affected spot.

These poultices are of great service for open sores on the feet: they hinder decomposition of the blood and putrid flesh.

Fœnum græcum can be bought of any apothecary.

Gentian, Yellow (*Gentiana lutea*, L.)

The gentian grows by preference on the mountains. Reliable persons may be sent to gather this inexpensive and excellent medicinal herb for you. First and foremost, I advise to prepare extract of gentian. For this purpose gentian roots must be well dried, chopped up small, and placed in bottles, into which pure spirits are poured.

This extract is the best stomachic. Twenty to thirty drops in six to eight table-spoonfuls of water is the dose, which may be taken daily for a considerable time. A good digestion and an excellent appetite will not fail soon to declare themselves. If we feel a weight on the stomach, as of imperfectly digested food, a tea-spoonful of gentian extract in half a glass of warm water will speedily remove the sensation.

It is wise to take a bottle of gentian extract in travelling. A few drops of it, taken on sugar when we are overtired or badly nourished, will render good service.

Nausea and fainting fits may be counteracted by a tea-spoonful of the tincture taken in water: it warms and revives, restoring peace alike to mind and body.

Gentian tea is similar in its effects. It is made by boiling the chopped up root or the gentian powder.

Honey.

There used to be a prejudice against allowing young people to eat honey; it was only good for the old, we were told by a former generation.

I have employed and tested honey in manifold ways, and always found it to be excellent in its effects. It loosens, purges, and strengthens.

Mixed with tea for catarrhs and conglutinations it is in general use.

The country people often make use of a honey ointment for healing boils. Whoever does not possess the proper knowledge for treating boils with cold water should have recourse to honey, rather than attempt to smear with any doubtful sort of grease. The honey ointment is easy to prepare, being simply composed of honey and white flour in equal parts, with a little water added to produce the right consistency. It should be tolerably stiff, not over liquid.

As internal medicine, honey is also of good service in many little complaints. Small tumours in the stomach are readily contracted and healed by means of honey; yet would I not advise to take the honey pure, but rather mixed with some suitable tea infusion.

For painful swallowing, in consequence of catarrh or sore throat, a tea-spoonful of honey boiled up in half a pint of water is the best and safest remedy. This will also be an excellent gargle for public singers who wish to clear their voice. This same mixture may furthermore be used for sore eyes, to which it is applied by means of a linen rag.

I know an old gentleman of eighty who prepares for himself his daily wine, consisting of a spoonful of honey boiled up in water. "My health and strength at this advanced age," he said to me, "I owe to the virtue of the honey wine." May be! So much at least I know from personal experience—for I have prepared much honey wine with my own hands, have seen it much drunk, and have now and then drunk a glass of it myself—that honey wine is purifying, nourishing, and strengthening in its effects. It always reminds me of the honey mead which our German forefathers used to drink, to which potent beverage they used to ascribe their strength and long life, as Tacitus tells us. Whoever feels inclined to imitate his ancestors in this respect, may find the recipe for brewing this obsolete drink at the end of this part.

HYPERCON (*Hypericum perforatum*, L.)

Hypercon, or St John's wort, used to be called *Hexenkraut* (witches' or magic herb) on account of its wonderful effects. Nowadays both the herb and its properties are alike forgotten.

This medicinal herb has particular influence upon the liver, and is best administered in the shape of tea. A slight admixture of aloe powder will heighten the effect, which may be traced by the blotches of clouded unhealthy matter which come away with the urine.

Headaches which proceed from watery matter or conglutination in the head, or from ascending gases, stomach pressure, slight conglutination of chest and lungs, may all be speedily cured by hypercon tea.

Mothers, to whom their little bed-wetters have caused much trouble and anxiety, have often had occasion to verify the strengthening effects of this tea.

In default of hypercon, milfoil (*Achilleia millefolium*, L.) may be employed for all the above-mentioned complaints.

JUNIPER (*Juniperus communis*, L.)

Who does not know the juniper-berry? Employed for fumigating purposes it diffuses a pleasant aromatic scent throughout rooms and corridors, and improves the atmosphere. I am no friend of fumigation in general, with sugar, vinegar, and suchlike, not comprehending what benefit the air derives from this practice. When, however, it is necessary to disinfect a room where infectious illness prevails, or where a corpse is present, no better means can be found than fumigations of juniper for dispersing and annihilating all floating poisonous germs and particles.

Its effects on our internal organism are of the same kind. These berries, so to say, fumigate the mouth and stomach, and arm us against infection. Those who nurse or attend on patients attacked with scarlet fever, smallpox, typhus, cholera, &c., should daily chew from six to ten of these berries. They will produce a pleasant taste in the mouth, and render good service to the digestion.

People whose stomach is weak should practise the following small juniper cure, the good effects of which have often been tested: the first day they should begin with four berries, the second day five berries, on the third day six, on the fourth day seven berries, and so on till twelve days and fifteen berries have been reached; after this go on diminishing the dose by one berry every day, till the portion has been reduced to five berries. I know many persons whose weakened and gas-overloaded stomachs have been cleansed and strengthened by this simple berry cure.

For stone and gravel, kidney and liver complaints, the juniper-berry has always stood in good repute since olden times; also in cases where it is necessary to secrete indolent gases, watery and slimy matter from the system.

Besides the berries, young sprouts of juniper may be employed for tea in the first stages of dropsy, likewise for purifying the blood.

Oil of juniper is best purchased in the apothecary's.

The tincture of juniper any one can make for himself, preparing it with wine, brandy, or other spirits.

KNOT-GRASS (*Polygonum aviculare*).

This plant, which does not seem to have been originally included in Pfarrer Kneipp's Pharmacy, has, however, quite recently been employed by the author with marked success in gravel and stone complaints (*see* Gravel). It is drunk as tea, which is infused in the manner repeatedly described.—Translator's note.

LAVENDER, OIL OF.

Lavender-oil can be procured at any apothecary's. It should never be wanting in the household pharmacy.

Five drops on sugar taken twice daily will improve the digestion and promote appetite.

Flatulency, headache occasioned by ascending gases, and nausea, may be relieved by this medicament.

For mental affections I have frequently employed

oil of lavender with success; and I maintain that the cure of such complaints is often effected by the removal of unhealthy gases in the brain region. In my opinion far too little importance is generally attached to the action of these gases. Those who suffer from flatulency know best what discomfort is caused them internally.

LIME (*Tilia grandifolia* and *parvifolia*, Ehrh.)

Only old people collect the once favourite blossoms of the lime-tree nowadays. They do right in being thus conservative.

Lime-blossom tea is, after the elder-flower tea, the best infusion for promoting perspiration. I am not a friend of artificially produced perspiration as generally practised, but I make frequent use of these flowers for the vapour applications which in my system take the place of sweating.

The effect of this tea is excellent in old neglected coughs, conglutination of lungs and windpipe, and in complaints of the abdomen which have their source in conglutination of the kidneys. In place of lime-blossom I sometimes make use of hypercon, with or without an admixture of milfoil.

LINSEED.

Linseed poultices are in general use, and require no explanation. With these, similar results may be achieved to those of fenugreek. I give the preference however to the latter, as it attacks the foe with greater force and energy.

MALLOW (*Althea rosea*, L.)

The mallow should not be absent from any flower-garden. The bountiful Creator, in laying on the colours of this pretty flower, has poured a drop of healing elixir into each tiny chalice.

Mallow blossoms, especially those of the black mallow, infused as tea, are good for throat complaints and loose conglutination of the chest.

Mallow is usually mixed with flowers of the great mullein.

Employed as vapour applications, mallow flowers are of great service for inhalations and for ear complaints.

MARSH-CLOVER (*Menyanthes trifoliata*, L.)

The marsh-clover is a plant which frequently grows in the neighbourhood of running water. In places where the stream, finding no issue, has poured itself into marshy spots inland, the marsh-clover will be found. It has three leaves, and is excellent for stomach and digestion; made into extract with brandy or spirits, it will likewise do good service.

MARSH-MALLOW (*Althea officinalis*, L.)

Tea of marsh-mallow, though much employed for cold and catarrhs, is no particular friend of mine. I have found it to be of uncertain or weak effect, and its slimy nature is apt to impair or destroy the appetite. To put it mildly, I find both root and herb of marsh-mallow to be of suspicious character. I never prescribe it to my patients, choosing instead such plants upon whose service I can rely.

MINT (*Mentha piperita*, L., and *Mentha aquatica*, L.)

Peppermint and watermint are both useful, and differ but little in their effects. I give the preference to watermint, being the more vigorous of the two. Mint is one of the most potent stomachics we know of: its scent alone reveals to us that it must possess no common virtues.

Leaves of mint bound about the brow in cases of severe headache will bring speedy relief.

A cupful of mint-tea, taken morning and evening, promotes digestion and gives a fresh healthy appearance to the face.

The same service may be rendered by the powder, of which I prescribe one to two pinches daily, taken in water or mixed with the food.

Persons who are much weakened after an illness, those who suffer from palpitation, from nausea, and from frequent and obstinate fits of vomiting, should often make use of both tea and powder.

A cupful of mint-tea infused with a mixture of wine-and-water will, if taken several days in succession, remove foul-smelling breath.

Decoction of mint prepared with vinegar, and taken from time to time in one to two tea-spoonfuls, will arrest blood spitting and vomiting.

Mint boiled in milk, and drunk warm, will relieve pain in the abdomen.

Let every housewife accord to this noble plant a corner in her garden alongside of the rue! It will amply reward her trouble, if only by the aromatic perfume which it so freely sheds around.

Misletoe (*Viscum album*, L.)

This parasite plant, which specially thrives upon old trees, possesses valuable medicinal qualities. Its healing powers are principally directed to the blood, and I cannot too strongly advise mothers to make early acquaintance with this herb.

Bloody flux is arrested by tea of misletoe. I could name a number of cases in which a single cupful sufficed to relieve the patient.

For other disorders of the circulation counsel may also be sought of the misletoe and its perfectly harmless tea.

Misletoe may be mixed with shave-grass in equal quantities, likewise with santala. (See Saunders.)

Mullein (*Verbascum Schraderi*, Meyer).

The flowers of the greater and of the lesser mullein are carefully collected by the peasants. They know that with these they can prepare an excellent gargle and a still more efficacious tea, which may be employed for throat complaints, catarrhs, conglutination of the chest, and difficulty in breathing.

Let me warmly recommend this tea. I usually mix the blossoms of mullein with those of the black mallow in equal quantities. This mixture is of more potent and durable effect than when the mullein is used alone.

Nettle (*Urtica dioica*, L.)

The most despised of all plants is the nettle. Some persons of supersensitive nature feel wounded by the mere mention of its name. Is this reasonable? I was lately rejoiced to hear that a schoolmaster — in Bohemia, I believe—had written a whole pamphlet on the subject of nettles; and in truth, for the initiated, the nettle is of inestimable value.

Fresh nettle leaves, dried and made into tea, serve to loosen conglutination in chest and lungs, and cleanse the stomach of superfluous matter, by secreting it through the urine.

Of yet more potent effect than leaves is the nettle root, either employed green in summer, or dried for winter use. Beginning dropsy may be arrested by nettle-root tea, which has the effect of thoroughly purifying the system from all indolent and unhealthy saps.

Those whose blood is impure should often, in summer, partake of nettles prepared as spinach. In Italy herb soups are in great favour. Herb *Knödel*[1] of nettles put in the soup are not only nourishing but medicinal.

Long sufferers from rheumatism, who have found all other means unavailing, should daily rub or flog the affected parts for some minutes with a bunch of fresh nettles. Fear of the unaccustomed rod will quickly give place to joy at its salutary effects.

Oak Bark.

What! Are we also to use oak bark as medicine? Yes, undoubtedly, either in fresh or dried shape.

The bark of young oak-trees boiled for half an hour

[1] The *Knödel*, for which no English synonym exists, is a round ball of dumpling consistency, the size of a small apple. There are many varieties of *Knödels*, sweet and savoury, some of the latter of which are boiled and eaten in soup.

produces a strong decoction. Dip into this a small towel and wind it round your neck. For all complaints in which the neck is unnaturally distended, when the glands are swollen, and in the beginning of goitre, it will render good service.

Whoever suffers from irritation of the rectum should take sitz-baths with oak-bark decoction; small injections of the same will assist the cure by dissolving the inconvenient and frequently dangerous fistulas.

Hard boils which are not inflamed, may likewise be treated with oak-bark decoction.

Oak-bark tea, like resin, has an invigorating effect on the internal organs.

OATS (*Avena sativa*, L.)

Thorough boiling serves to extract the inward essence of oats (essence of barley may be produced in the same way). This beverage is nourishing, easily digested, and cooling: it is of good effect in interior heats, and very nourishing for convalescents who are much weakened in consequence of smallpox, typhus, and suchlike illnesses. How often do I regret that these poor creatures, who stand above all in want of being provided with a fresh supply of blood, are denied this valuable elixir, while every other imaginable kind of beverage is given to them!

Its preparation is simple: one quart of oats are washed six to eight times in fresh cold water, then boiled in two quarts of water until the liquid is reduced by one-half. Into the strained liquid mix two spoonfuls of honey, and let the mixture boil up again for a few minutes.

Regulating Purgative.

Forty or fifty years ago people were in the habit of having themselves bled at some particular annual date, usually determined by the moon; and at certain other yearly or half-yearly dates to take a violent purgative. Even nowadays there are many who cling to the delusion that a radical clearing out of the system should be undertaken from time to time.

I am diametrically opposed to all such violent measures, being of opinion that the same results may be achieved by mild and harmless means.

For long I have searched among the plants, probing the qualities of those which seemed to me most likely to be of beneficial effect on the digestion. At last I have succeeded in discovering two different combinations of herbs which, in their united strength—"viribus unitis"—will produce the desired result.

The two recipes, of which I make no secret, are as follows:—

Regulating Purgative No. I.

2 table-spoonfuls ground fennel.
2 table-spoonfuls crushed juniper-berries.
1 table-spoonful powdered aloe.
1 table-spoonful fenugreek.

Everything to be well mixed and kept in a dry spot.

The medicine, which acts only twelve to thirty hours after it has been taken, is boiled as tea for a quarter of an hour. One tea-spoonful of the mixture will suffice for a small cupful of tea, to be taken hot or cold, with or without sugar, by the patient at bedtime.

Very strong and robust persons may take a cup of this tea two days in succession.

Weaker patients will do better to divide the one cupful over two or three days, so as to take from four to six table-spoonfuls every evening.

Many who take this tea will be disappointed at obtaining no results, although they be conscious of a lively rumbling and working in the interior. The police sometimes search in vain when there are no delinquents to be discovered. The regulating purgative does likewise, and when it finds no unhealthy matter to be removed, it forbears to weaken the system by unnecessary purging.

This tea is also of particular effect on the urine, and has often served to remove considerable conglutinations on the chest.

Regulating Purgative No. II.

The second recipe for the preparation of the purgative is as follows:—

2 table-spoonfuls ground fennel.
3 table-spoonfuls crushed juniper-berries.
3 table-spoonfuls danewort root powder.
1 table-spoonful fenugreek.
1 table-spoonful powder of aloe.

The tea, which does not necessarily act as a laxative, is principally intended to influence the kidneys and bladder, whose unhealthy matter it secretes through the urine. Those who are conscious of discomfort in the abdomen (in the neighbourhood of the bladder), of burning pain in bladder or kidneys, and of difficulty in making water, may fearlessly employ this medicine, which is also useful in the first stages of dropsy.

Its application is the same as the foregoing.

Resin.

As the candle sometimes drips, so likewise does it drip from the stems of pine and fir trees. Any one who goes to the forest in summer or autumn can mark how the liquid sap wells out of the trunk. Like tears suspended against the tree-stem, are these resin-drops, white as wax, clear as honey, fresh as spring-water.

This resin is the pine-tree's blood, and when the tree receives a deep wound it bleeds profusely.

Five to six of the resin drops or tears, swallowed daily for some length of time, will strengthen the chest, and fortify the internal organs.

As a substitute for resin-drops, for those who do not live in the vicinity of pine-forests, grains of white incense may be used. Six to eight of these grains taken daily will be a good chest-cure.

Let none be afraid of these resin-pills, for they are easily digested.

Ribwort (*Plantago lanceolata*, L.)

When a peasant happens to wound himself over his field labour, he quickly seeks out the ribwort; squeezing and pressing the stiff stubborn leaf till he has extracted from it some drops of juice. This valuable sap he either applies direct to the spot, or else moistens with it a linen rag, with which the wound is bandaged.

Should the leaf prove obstinate, and only produce a slight moisture, then the leaf itself should be applied bodily to the affected part. This bandage is the simplest, and often the best of all others. As with golden threads, the ribwort sews together the edges of the gaping wound; and like pure gold, which does not admit of the presence of rust, so too the ribwort averts corruption and decomposition of flesh and blood.

The internal effects of this plant are no less noteworthy. If only hundreds of suffering individuals would but collect these leaves in spring and summer, express and drink their healing sap! By this simple means many complaints which have their origin in impure blood might be averted.

Dried leaves of ribwort likewise produce an excellent tea, most efficacious for internal conglutination.

Many a one buys ribwort in the apothecary's for hard cash. Good peasant! be thou thine own collector, distiller, and apothecary. At least thou canst be sure of having the genuine article.

A mixture of dried ribwort and lungwort (*Pulmonaria officinalis*) leaves, in equal quantities, is often very effective.

ROSE-HIPS (*Rosa canina*, L.)

A thoughtful mother will not merely pluck the flower of the dogrose bush, but, mindful of the household pharmacy, she will also collect the hips, which may be employed not only for sauces and jams, but likewise as medicaments. She will lay in the greater supply of these if a member of her family be afflicted with kidney, stone, or gravel complaint. Rose-hip tea serves to purify both kidneys and bladder.

When the seeds have been removed from the hips, the berry is dried, and is thus employed as tea.

Rosemary (*Rosmarinus officinalis*, L.)

No wedding guest should be without a nosegay of this flower, and it were a shame if the herb-collector forgot to pluck it for the household pharmacy.

Rosemary is an excellent stomachic. Prepared and drunk as tea, it cleanses the stomach from slime and conglutination, restores appetite and digestion. The dose is from two to four table-spoonfuls, taken morning and evening.

Rosemary wine taken in small portions is useful in heart complaints. It acts as a sedative, and when dropsy of the heart exists, secretes the water through the urine.

For dropsy in general, rosemary wine may be taken with good effect.

In either case, three to four table-spoonfuls of this wine, which is of very pleasant taste, taken morning and evening, will be the proper dose.

Rosemary wine is prepared by chopping up small a handful of rosemary and placing it in a bottle, into which is then poured pure white wine, which should not be too new. Red wine may also be used, but white is preferable. Half a day will suffice to render this rosemary wine ready for use. It should be strained clear of the leaves, which can be used a second time by pouring fresh wine over them.

Rue (*Ruta graveolens*, L.)

The properties of this noble medicinal herb are unfortunately too little known or appreciated. Scent is the language of plants. How distinctly and impressively does not the rue declare its goodwill to help us, to relieve our pain and suffering! It speaks as eloquently as though each tiny leaf were a little tongue. Would that we always understood this language!

However and wherever the rue is applied, it is of strengthening and invigorating effect.

If we only chew one little leaf, we quickly recognise its virtues. A refreshing aromatic taste will pervade the mouth, like incense perfume throughout a house.

For congestions, headache, giddiness, the tea of rue is excellent, and no less so in all cases of hysteria, palpitations, difficulty in breathing, and all cramp-like complaints of the abdomen.

Expressed in brandy or spirits, extract of rue may be taken instead of tea, the dose—which should on no account be exceeded—being from ten to twelve drops on sugar twice daily.

Oil of rue is taken in the same fashion. It is prepared by putting dried rue-leaves in a glass, and pouring over them fine salad-oil, after which the glass must be allowed to stand in a warm place for a considerable length of time. Afterwards, when strained, it will be ready for use.

SAGE (*Salvia officinalis*, L.)

In laying out a new garden, do not forget the sage; it is a pretty ornamental plant. I have often seen how a passer-by will pluck a sage leaf to rub with it his black or discoloured teeth. This sufficiently demonstrates the cleansing power of this plant.

Old suppurated wounds, washed and poulticed with a decoction of sage, will quickly heal.

Conglutination in the gums, stomach, or throat are cured by sage-tea.

Sage, prepared as tea, with a mixture of wine and water, purifies the kidneys and liver.

More potent effects may be achieved if sage be mixed in equal proportions with wormwood.

Reduced to powder, and strewn over the food like salt or pepper, sage will render the same services as when it is infused as tea.

SALAD-OIL.

Read the remarks under the heading of almond-oil, for only in default of, or in conjunction with, the former, is salad-oil to be employed. By salad-oil I understand pure olive-oil, or at the very least unadulterated oil of reps.

SAUNDERS (*Santala,* see MISLETOE).

Saunders is a red powder usually employed for dyeing purposes, which can be purchased of any apothecary.

I invariably mix this perfectly harmless medicament with misletoe-tea in the proportion of one table-spoonful of misletoe-leaves to two pinches of santala. The tea thus prepared is of stronger effect than tea of misletoe alone.

SAUERKRAUT OR PICKLED CABBAGE (*Brassica oleracea capitata,* L.)

This (in Germany) well-known domestic remedy deserves to be mentioned here.

For wounds, burns, and similar accidents, in great heats, for dissolving and secreting ancient evils, &c.,

fresh-plucked cabbage-leaves applied to the affected spot or limb will render excellent service.

It is of inestimable value for country people, the more so for being always close at hand and easily procured.

In the third part of this book the reader will be able to see for himself how and where the sauerkraut is employed.

Secretive Oil.

There are cases in which so much unhealthy matter is contained in the body that it is very difficult to dissolve and secrete these poisonous germs. This difficulty does not consist in the water's insufficient action, but is rather to be ascribed to the patient himself, whose debility and infirmity of purpose often causes him to shrink from the prospect of a prolonged course of treatment.

I pondered long over this question, when it occurred to me that outward eruptions have frequently had the effect of expelling unhealthy matter from the interior.

My researches were therefore directed to the discovery of some means of artificially producing an outward rash or eruption, which would assist and curtail the cold water's operation.

After long seeking, I hit upon an oil which fulfils these conditions. Its effect is perfectly harmless but thorough, and it is only used as an external medicine.

A few examples may serve to illustrate the action of this remedy.

Somebody, for instance, complains of sore eyes; the eyes are red and sensitive to the light, watery matter drops from them, and the pain is considerable.

In such cases I first rub the skin behind the ear gently, to produce slight warmth, and then apply three or four drops of oil to the spot. In half an hour the patient will be conscious of the effect by a feeling of distension and burning. In twenty-four hours numerous small fistules filled with water will have appeared at the place. These will subsequently dry up and disappear. Should the first application not succeed—viz., not produce an effect, after an interval of thirty hours—it may be repeated on the following day. I have successfully cured many eye complaints by this means.

Violent toothache afflicts another patient; the gums are swollen, the jaw painful, the whole head affected. As in the former case, I rub a few drops of this oil behind the ear, or at the nape of the neck. The effect is certain.

One peculiarity of this oil is that the irritation and soreness of the skin produced by its first application, is completely cured by the second one.

I do not in the least regard this medicine as a secret remedy, and have disclosed its composition to many trusty friends. In order, however, to preclude any abuse in its employment, I am for the present prevented from publishing the receipe.

SHAVE-GRASS (*Equisetum arvense*, L.)

I cannot sufficiently praise the manifold and excellent qualities of this herb. It is not merely useful for cleansing all kitchen vessels, for which reason it is much prized by every housewife, but likewise it serves to purify and heal internal and external complaints of the human body.

For old suppurated wounds, even those of a cancerous nature, it is of remarkable effect. It cleans, dissolves, and, so to say, scarifies the unhealthy matter. This herb is either employed as decoction for lavations, swathings, compresses, or else the leaves themselves placed between damp cloths are applied to the affected part: as a vapour application it is likewise valuable in particular cases.

Taken as internal medicine the shave-grass is of still greater value.

Shave-grass tea, which can harm no one, purifies the stomach. A cupful of this taken occasionally (not daily) will be of good effect. It assuages the pains in stone and gravel complaints, and is of special service in promoting urine, for patients who suffer from difficulty in water-making. Directions as to its application for this complaint will be found under the head of diseases.

For bloody flux and blood-spitting, it is one of the best and most effective teas.

Violent bleeding of the nose may be rapidly stilled by drawing up the infusion through the nostrils.

A plentiful supply of shave-grass should be wanting in no household pharmacy.

SILVERWEED (*Potentilla anserina*, L.)

This plant, as indicated by its Latin name, grows oftenest where flocks of geese are wont to feed. It may likewise be found near cottages, in the fields, or by the side of the brook. Many people call it the "cramp herb" because of its effects.

Tea of silverweed is an excellent remedy for fits of cramp, whether in the stomach or abdomen. Even in cases of spasm and tetanus, it has frequently been of good service. When the fits begin to appear, or, better still, when the first approaching symptoms have been detected, let the patient take thrice daily boiled milk (as warm as possible), in which a large pinch—as much as can be grasped with three fingers—of this herb has been cooked.

To intensify the effect, compresses dipped in an infusion of the herb may simultaneously be applied to the affected parts.

SLOE (*Prunus spinosa*, L.)

Sloe-blossoms are the most harmless laxative, and should be wanting in no household pharmacy.

Boil up sloe-blossoms for one minute, and daily drink a cupful of this tea during three to four days. It will act gently and painlessly, but at the same time thoroughly.

As a cleansing and strengthening stomachic, I can also warmly recommend this tea.

STRAWBERRY (*Fragaria vesca*, L.)

How delighted are the children when they can bring the first bunch of strawberries to their parents, pastor, or schoolmaster! With what rejoicing is the first dish of this refreshing fruit placed on the table as dessert in every house!

Not only the fruit but also the strawberry-leaves are generally beloved. Many a mother returning homewards after a hard day's labour gathers these leaves for her sickly child, well knowing this strawberry-leaf tea to be one of the cheapest, most wholesome, and nourishing beverages.

How is this tea prepared? Take of the (dried) strawberry-leaves as much as you can grasp in three to four fingers, pour half a pint of boiling water upon them, and carefully cover the jar or pot. After five minutes strain off the infusion, and mix with a little milk and sugar.

Woodruff (*Asperula odorata,* L.) mixed with the strawberry-leaves, in the proportion of one-quarter or one-third, will give more body and flavour to the tea.

Fresh perfect strawberry-leaves, collected in May or June at sunny spots, more especially on high hill slopes, will produce an excellent beverage.

The medicinal qualities of the berries themselves are not to be despised. They should be given freely to all convalescents who are much debilitated after severe illness: half a pint of milk mixed with a gill of strawberries taken daily—or else twice a-day, a gill of strawberries, eaten with a good piece of rye-bread—will do excellent service, and tend not only to strengthen the system, but likewise to purify the blood. In winter, strawberry-jam will produce almost the same effects.

Great internal heat in summer, even in cases of high fever, may easily be relieved by a plate of strawberries.

Strawberries taken daily are good for gravel and stone complaints. The same remark applies to liver complaints and to skin eruptions produced by an impure state of the blood. For these complaints as much as two pints may be taken daily, morning and evening.

SUCCORY, WILD (*Cichorium intybus,* L.)

This plant, called in German *Wegwart* (literally,

waiting on the way), will be found by the roadside waiting patiently to be plucked for the household pharmacy. It is also called turnsole, because it ever turns its leaves towards the sun. The succory has an untidy rough appearance, like an unkempt child among its neater comrades. Its blue flower alone, somewhat paler than the corn-flower, raises its position, and inspires a certain amount of respect.

Appearances are often deceitful, and so it is with the wild succory, which, under a rough exterior, bears a golden heart.

Tea of succory-leaves dissolves conglutination of the stomach, and secretes gall and bile. It purifies liver, kidneys, and milt, and secretes unhealthy matter through the urine. The dose is two cupfuls daily, taken morning and evening, during three to four days.

Pains and inflammation of the stomach may be relieved by compresses dipped in a hot infusion of succory leaves and flowers, renewed two to three times.

Chicory-leaves may be expressed in spirits, which will serve to rub consumptive or dwindling limbs two to three times daily.

As leaves and blossoms, so also the roots may be employed for the same purposes. These are easiest dug up in rainy weather.

VALERIAN (*Valeriana officinalis*, L.)

The innate strength of valerian is proved to us by its effect upon cats, which it stupefies to the extent of causing them to roll in it.

We make use of the root only, which, chopped up and infused as tea, or ground to powder, may be taken in small doses.

Valerian root has much the same effect as rue in relieving headache and cramp-like complaints, by expelling unwholesome gases.

VIOLET (*Viola odorata,* L.)

The perfume of this sweet-scented spring flower should also pervade our household pharmacy.

For spring coughs in children let the anxious mother take a handful of green or dried violet-leaves (the root bruised, chopped up, may likewise be employed), and having boiled it as tea, administer it in doses of two to three spoonfuls, at intervals of from two to three hours.

In consumption, it likewise relieves the cough and assists the process of dissolving slime and conglutination.

The dose in these cases is from three to five tablespoonfuls, at intervals of from two to three hours.

This tea serves, furthermore, for headaches and great heat in the head.

The head may either be completely washed with the violet tea, or else linen bandages dipped in the infusion may be bound about the patient's head.

It is an excellent gargle for inflamed throat, and may also serve to moisten a linen compress, which should be wound tightly round the neck.

Difficulty in breathing, having its origin in unhealthy gases of the bowels and abdomen, may be relieved by drinking daily two large, or three small, cupfuls of violet tea, and continuing this cure for a considerable length of time.

Violet-leaves, bruised and applied to inflamed boils,

will cool and relieve; boiled in vinegar, their decoction is efficacious for gout.

WORMWOOD (*Artemisia absinthium*, L.)

Wormwood is one of the best known stomachics. It secretes wind, improves and strengthens the stomach saps, and produces appetite, whether prepared as tea or in the shape of powder.

For foul-smelling breath, wormwood is of excellent effect.

Those who suffer from the liver (melancholy) may take one to two pinches daily of wormwood powder, mixed in a spoonful of soup, or strewed over the food like salt or pepper. The patient's jaundiced complexion will rapidly give place to a healthy colour.

Wormwood may also be prepared as tincture, and can be kept for years without deterioration. A single leaf of wormwood is sufficient to impart a bitter taste to a whole bottle of spirits.

Travellers prone to stomach disorders should never set out on a journey without this trusty friend and companion.

Wormwood tea has frequently done good service as an eye-water for sore or inflamed eyes.

APPENDIX.

Recipe for Making Bran Bread.

The wheat should be ground in the mill along with the bran; care must be taken in order to ensure this, as the miller is likely to object to the proceeding.

Of this bran-flour take from 2 to 8 lb. (according to the quantity of bread required) in a dish, and mix with warm water till the right consistency. Place overnight in a moderately warm spot. Neither yeast, salt, nor other seasoning should enter into its composition.

On the following day small oval loaves or rolls are formed of the paste, and are put to bake in a moderately hot oven from an hour and a quarter to an hour and a half.

When removed from the oven, the baked bread should be plunged in boiling water from three to four minutes, until the whole loaves or rolls be thoroughly penetrated with the moisture, after which they are again replaced in the oven until completely dry. This last proceeding was taught to me by the prior of a Trappist convent, who, after having tried various methods, selected this one as the best for extracting the nutritious properties of bran.

Many persons, who eat this bread in preference to any other, have told me that it is most efficacious in all stomach complaints, and especially for piles.

The bread should be kept in a cool place, and if the rind be too hard, wrapped in a moist linen cloth.

Recipe for Honey-wine or Mead.

The old Germans had little or no wine; our brown beer was unknown to them, because it did not yet exist. Their food was very simple, and yet they were a powerful race, long-lived and healthy. These qualities they ascribed to the use of mead. It is a pity that this noble beverage should be so little known to-day, replaced as it is by the general use of beer, often so adulterated as no longer to deserve the name of a wholesome beverage.

My recipe for preparing mead is as follows: Into a clean copper caldron I pour from 13 to 15 gallons of soft water. When this is pretty warm, about 5 quarts of honey are gradually stirred in. Water and honey together should be allowed to boil slowly for an hour and a half. From time to time t e impure froth should be skimmed off from the surface. .Vhen finished boiling, the honey-water is poured into tin or earthen vessels, and allowed to cool down to lukewarm heat, after which it is transferred to a carefully cleaned cask, which should be loosely plugged. If the cellar be moderately warm, it will begin to ferment after from five to ten days. When fourteen days have elapsed, the young honey-wine, poured clear of the dregs, is removed to a second cask. The second process of fermentation lasts from ten to fourteen days; and only then, when the mead has finally settled, and no further sounds are heard inside the cask, is the plug to be fixed in firmly. In three to four weeks the mead will be clear and ready for use. Drawn off into bottles, well corked and buried in cool sand, it will in a few days be very frothy. This beverage is cooling, and well adapted to fever patients who are unable to drink wine or beer. It is also a good drink for the healthy, but should only be imbibed in small portions, for taken in large quantities it is apt to produce disgust.

CONTENTS OF A SMALL HOUSEHOLD PHARMACY.

I. Extract of—

Arnica.
Bilberry.
Gentian.
Juniper-berries.
Rosemary.
Succory.
Wormwood.

II. Tea of—

Angelica.
Camomile.
Centaury.
Coltsfoot.
Cowslip.
Danewort.
Elder.
Eyebright.
Hypercon.
Juniper-berries.
Knot-grass.
Lime.
Mallow.
Marsh-clover.
Marsh-mallow.
Milfoil.
Mint.
Misletoe.
Mullein, greater.
Nettle.
Oak bark.
Regulating purgative.
Ribwort.
Rose-hips.
Rosemary.
Rue.
Sage.
Succory, wild.
Shave-grass.
Silverweed.
Sloe.
Strawberry.
Valerian.
Violet.
Woodruff.
Wormwood.

III. Powder of—

Aloe.
Alum.
Angelica.
Coltsfoot.
Danewort.
Eyebright.
Fennel.
Fenugreek.
Linseed.
Mint.
Sage.
Saunders (santala).
Valerian.
Wormwood.
Ashes.
Bone-dust.
Chalk.

IV. Oil of—

Almond.
Aniseed.
Camphor.
Clove.
Fennel.
Juniper.
Lavender.
Rue.
Salad.

PART III.

DISEASES

INTRODUCTION.

THE following cases are no imaginary or fictitious ones. They are, one and all, taken from life.

I am well aware that this third part is most defective and incomplete, and that it utterly fails in exhausting or even enumerating the various diseases to which we are prone. Want of time and space is partly answerable for this result, which, however, is likewise to a certain degree intentional.

As the gardener who gathers a nosegay does not pluck of each sort of flower in equal quantity, so have I also, in detailing the various diseases, principally dwelt upon those which seem to me to be most interesting and instructive.

Diseases are crosses, dear reader! Sooner or later each one of us will be called upon to carry such a cross, sometimes unto the grave. But a merciful Providence permits us to seek to lighten our burden —as already the prophet Elias, speaking to Naaman the Syrian leper prince, has said: "Go and wash seven times in the Jordan, and thy flesh shall recover health, and thou shalt be clean."

Abdomen, Conglutination of.

A gentleman came to me and related: "I have constantly great pains in the neighbourhood of the kidneys, so violent as sometimes to be almost unbearable. Various doctors whom I consulted pronounced it to be disease of the kidneys and enlargement of the abdomen. I suffer from nausea, headache, dizziness, acidity in the stomach; the urine is scanty; I am never without pains in the feet, and cannot stand for long. I have much perspiration and great weakness; my complexion is always unhealthy."

The patient had lost all courage, and because the medicinal remedies availed him nothing, he had recourse to water.

The applications which I prescribed were as follows: 1. Daily, two upper affusions and knee affusions; 2. Daily, one back affusion; and twice to three times daily walking in water or in wet grass. It being summer, the applications could be more lavishly made use of. Immense quantities of urine were secreted; the desire to vomit ceased upon the second day; the complexion improved, and with renewed strength so also new courage and life were regained. In fourteen days he was completely cured; had it not been summer, the course of treatment would perhaps have lasted fourteen days more.

Acidity.

Crescentia relates: "I am forty-five years old, and suffer almost daily from pains in the stomach. It stops from time to time, but only for short intervals.

I have frequently a sour and bitter taste in the mouth, and am almost always cold."

This person's appearance was very painful: the body emaciated, the features drawn. Defective digestion had evidently produced a great poverty of blood.

I prescribed as follows: Pour boiling water on hay-flowers; put these as hot as possible in a cloth or bag, which place on the stomach, as hot as you can bear it, and leave it there an hour and a half. Do this for three days; take every evening a warm foot-bath with ashes and salt—fourteen minutes on three consecutive days; then every third or fourth day rise from bed, and wash the body completely, returning to bed immediately. Do this also at night three or four times weekly. Then take twice daily from four to six spoonfuls of wormwood tea, and so on for fourteen days. After this one foot-bath a-week and one nightly washing will be sufficient.

Asthma.

A gentleman relates as follows: "I am forty-six years old. For twenty years I have suffered from asthma. I had recourse to various doctors, but they pronounced my disease to be incurable, and none of their remedies produced any effect. The difficulty in breathing was sometimes so great that even in winter I was obliged to stand by the open window in order not to choke. I had already given up all hope, and resigned myself to carry my cross into the grave. This condition sometimes lasted for several days consecutively, entailing great weakness and complete loss of appetite. At last God was merciful,—the book 'Meine Wasserkur' fell into my hands at the time of my greatest need.

Within a week I was completely cured. It is scarcely credible that water alone should suffice to reform nature in so short a space. The applications of which I made use were:—

"1. Upper affusion, followed by the knee affusion, walking in water.

"2. Back affusion, lower affusion.

"3. Sitz-bath, upper affusion, semi-bath.

"4. Upper affusion, back affusion.

"5. Semi-bath, upper affusion, sitz-bath.

"6. Complete bath, upper affusion.

"7. Lower affusion, upper affusion.

"In addition to this, for one to two hours walking barefoot in wet grass. This course of treatment I went through in summer, and day by day I felt relief."

Bed-wetting.

This complaint is of frequent occurrence among children of both sexes. Even among adults it is not uncommon. It is a grave error to try and cure children by means of corporal punishment, which mostly produces a directly opposite effect. Weakness of the system is the cause of this failing, which will readily disappear when the constitution has been strengthened and braced.

Six children, whose ages ranged from eight to thirteen years, were ordered by me to stand daily in cold water reaching up to the calves from three to five minutes, and then take exercise until the body had regained its normal temperature. After five days of this proceeding only two of the children had a relapse, and in a very few days more all were completely cured.

A second application consisted in holding the arms two minutes in water after each foot-bath, which tended to restore a healthy colour to their pale sickly faces.

Adults may employ these same means. Such only whose blood has been impoverished by debility should in addition take daily a cup of milfoil infusion, drinking the one half in the morning, the other half at night.

I must further remark that the coldest water is always the best for this purpose. I have tested the use of warm water with children, and have always achieved an opposite result.

BIRTH.

A young woman had given birth to three dead children: she was very sad and quite discouraged, the more so as the doctor had told her that she would never be able to produce a living child. I consoled her by saying that if she would have recourse to my cold-water applications, her system would be so strengthened as to be able eventually to bear pregnancy. To the poor despairing woman this sounded like a joyful revelation.

The treatment was begun with some of the very slightest applications for hardening and bracing the system, which were gradually increased in strength until she was able to stand whole and semi baths. Within the space of three years she presented three strong healthy children to the happy father.

A woman was ill with typhus; she suffered from terrible headaches. Her relations removed her from town to the country, in order that she might there die quietly. The poor woman was about to become a mother. I, being consulted, prescribed short wrappings, which were at once applied. The headache ceased. The patient's former doctor, being asked, pronounced that the first of these wrappings must infallibly have the effect of prematurely forcing on the confinement. In the meantime, however, six such wrappings had been applied without bad results. The patient recovered completely, and gave birth to a healthy child.

Bladder, Catarrh of the.

A gentleman relates: "I am thirty years old, and have now suffered over three years from this complaint, brought on by the retention of urine, necessitated by my employment. At first I struggled against the disease; but was at last obliged to give up my profession. Four months I lay ill in bed: my body had worn away till it almost resembled a skeleton; its weight was reduced to 82 lb. The doctor ordered me Wildung mineral waters, of which I drank almost one hundred bottles, and warm sitz-baths. In addition to the first illness, I got a violent catarrh of the stomach and bowels. In spring my strength somewhat rallied, only, however, to collapse anew when winter came."

The patient's appearance was most wretched and emaciated, but he had no cough. I gave him hopes of recovery. Already on the third day his complexion had improved, the pains decreased day by day, urination became easier and more plentiful, and in four weeks he declared, "Now I am once more the strong, healthy, and cheerful man I used to be. The water has done this."

The result in his case was indeed extraordinarily successful. A doctor, whose specialty it is to treat diseases of the bladder, pronounced the gentleman to be completely healed, and was quite surprised at the result.

The applications made use of were: At the beginning the patient had to sit several times on a vase over a steaming infusion of shave-grass; during three weeks, twice daily upper affusions and water-walking; later on, sitz-baths and upper affusion on alternate days, besides drinking an infusion of shave-grass and juniper-berries.

Bladder, Stone in the.

A gentleman in the prime of life fell ill. He had violent pains in the kidneys, and could not make water. The doctor declared that a stone was in the bladder, which could only be removed by an operation. To this, however, the patient would not consent.

To an acquaintance who came to see him the patient related his troubles. This friend advised him thrice a-day to take a warm sitz-bath of shave-grass, and before each bath to drink a cupful of shave-grass infusion. Within thirty-six hours a piece of stone nearly as large as a walnut had come out. The pain suddenly ceased, and the man was cured.

Blood, Decomposition of the.

Returning home from a mission, I went to visit a clergyman, having heard accidentally that his end was at hand. Entering, I found the reverend gentleman sitting in an arm-chair. He related: "I have twenty-five holes and wounds in my body. You see here on the face alone five plasters, and on the body there are twenty. Small boils containing a brown fluid appear suddenly, and when I remove the plaster after a day, small particles of putrid decomposed flesh are attached to it. I suffer in this fashion for months, and can find no relief. Still more unendurable than the wounds in the body, is the horrid nauseous taste in the mouth, which I cannot describe. Dear reverend colleague, if you know of any advice for a poor man, give it quickly, for it is high time."

I advised the unhappy patient to swallow, every two hours, from four to six spoonfuls of sage and wormwood infusion, in order to remove the nauseous taste from the mouth. Then I left him, expecting to see him again in the other world.

Five days later came a messenger, not bringing, however, the expected news of his decease, but with the joyful intelligence that the nauseous taste had disappeared and appetite was beginning to set in. As my first piece of advice had succeeded so well, I was begged to follow it up. I sent word that during fourteen days he was to wash the entire body daily with cold water as rapidly as possible. Again came the messenger to say the condition had improved and appetite was increasing. As further applications I then ordered during several weeks on alternate days a Spanish mantle, and a lavation of the entire body. Fourteen days after this he was able to say Mass again. For some time he continued to take weekly a bath of hay-flower 95° F., succeeded by a cold lavation. Also on alternate days a cold semi-bath, combined with upper affusion, and a lavation of the whole body. My reverend colleague completely recovered, and was able to practise his holy vocation twenty-four years longer to the end of his life.

Blood, Poisoning of the.

A woman had received a trifling injury to the finger, which might have been caused by a nail or wood-splinter. Disregarding this, she went to bed without examining the wound. In the night she was roused by a violent and painful cramp in the finger, accompanied by nausea. The wound was on the left hand, and she experienced also cramp and pain in the right leg. Within ten hours the hand swelled up to the elbow, became dark-red in hue, and the pain grew unbearable. There was no doctor in the village, and the case was urgent, as the blood-poisoning was spreading rapidly.

For eight consecutive hours the hand and arm were poulticed completely in hay-flowers infused in boiling water, and applied as hot as could be endured. By this means the spreading poison was arrested. An hour or two later she could not have been saved, for already the tongue had been affected. After thirty-six hours, the swelling had so relaxed that the skin hung like an empty bag over the flesh. As the cramps in the finger ceased, so also the pain and sickness disappeared.

Blood, Poverty of the.

Good and sufficient blood is indispensable to perfect health ; air, light, exercise, and proper nourishment are the means by which this end is attained. When one or other of these conditions is wanting, then the blood deteriorates in quantity or in quality.

Poverty of blood may also proceed from losing blood through wounds, leeches, or by the lancet.

Those who suffer from green - sickness, as this malady is called, present a distressing picture: their face is pale, sometimes yellow or brown; lips and gums especially are bloodless; the eyelids heavy; the carriage stooping and dejected; the body emaciated. Palpitation, difficulty in breathing, headache, pains in the back, impediments in the digestion, cramps, and faintings are some of its frequent consequences, Such persons are often affected with a diseased craving for unwholesome and unnatural food.

Fresh air and light clothing are the first rules to be observed in order to effect a cure, along with good, easily digestible food: milk, pure bread and bread soup, along with simple farinaceous preparations. Not much should be eaten at a time; two to four table-spoonfuls of milk taken frequently will have the best results, for, the stomach saps being weakened, digestion acts but slowly. Moderate exercise in the open air should be taken, without, however, overtaxing the powers.

The water applications are as follows: Three to four times weekly let the patient rise from bed, and having washed the whole body, return there quickly; standing in water up to the calves for one minute, succeeded by holding the arms in water two to three times weekly.

If the patient be much weakened and possessed of little latent heat, the water should at first be applied warm, and mixed with salt or vinegar. To incite the appetite, two to three table-spoonfuls of wormwood infusion, taken thrice daily, will be found useful. An excellent remedy against green-sickness is likewise a pinch of powdered chalk in four to six spoonfuls of water twice daily.

When the general tone of the system has been raised, then the foot-bath and lavations can be replaced by semi-baths two to three times weekly; and these again ultimately exchanged for upper and knee affusions applied in moderation.

Blood, Spitting or Vomiting.

When blood appears, it is important to ascertain whether this proceeds from the stomach or the lungs. Blood from the lungs may be mostly recognised by being thrown up with cough, and by its frothy pale-red appearance; while blood from the stomach is usually dark-red or coffee-brown, and hangs together in clumps and masses. Blood-spitting is always alarming, and requires caution, as it may be attended with more or less danger.

If the blood proceed from the stomach, who can tell which little vein has suffered, and when the bleeding may not be repeated? Neglect of these symptoms may bring about poverty of blood, or other severe complaints. If the cause be speedily ascertained and cured, then the stomach-bleeding will entail no further consequences.

More important and ominous by far is bleeding from the lungs. No time should be lost in setting this to rights.

Infusion of shave-grass is useful in both cases, because of its astringent properties. If blood has come through the nose, let the patient frequently draw up the infusion through the nostrils. If it comes from the mouth, the same infusion taken in spoonfuls every few minutes will be efficacious. This remedy sometimes acts very quickly in arresting the bleeding; but even after this has completely ceased, the proceeding should be continued for some time. In my personal experience, this infusion of shave-grass has never failed to bring about the desired result.

Should, however, the bleeding prove obstinate and of frequent recurrence, then its cause must be carefully examined into. Either the lung itself is directly affected, or else there is excessive determination of blood to the head (see Congestions), or it may have its origin in tumours of the stomach.

I do not speak here of hæmorrhage, which, resulting from injury to some important artery, is often fatal. All help is mostly here of no avail.

A word here as to nose-bleeding. Many persons bleed frequently from the nose without attaching much importance to the circumstance, the more so as they usually experience relief. Nevertheless this condition is an unhealthy one, which sooner or later must pave the way to serious illness. Independently of all other considerations, this proceeding, if of frequent recurrence, must produce poverty of blood, with all its attendant evils, such as alarm, nervous tremors, and depression.

The principal object to be aimed at in all such cases seems to me to restore regular circulation, by leading down the superfluous blood to the body and extremities, which are mostly found to be cold and bloodless.

A warm foot-bath mixed with salt and ashes, employed two to three times a-week for fifteen minutes, will prove an excellent medium, accompanied by walking two to three times weekly on wet stones, and as often a short swathing. When Nature has partially regained her strength, the upper and lower affusions, along with semi-baths and lavations of the upper body, may be resorted to.

One sort of nose-bleeding there is which is not only ominous, but sometimes directly fatal. I was once called in to administer the last sacraments to a young girl sixteen years of age, apparently in a dying condition, who, within the space of one and a half hour, had lost three basinfuls of blood through the nose. All household remedies had been tried in vain, and no doctor was to be had. I speedily ordered the contents of half a watering-can to be poured over her head, the other half over her back. The bleeding stopped immediately. The girl lay for several hours quite quiet, but more or less unconscious from weakness. Hardly had she revived a little when the nose-bleeding returned. The proceeding with the watering-can repeated, had the same effect as before, and the patient's strength was kept up by means of milk administered in spoonfuls half-hourly. In two days she was able to swallow soup, and within a few days a healthy appetite had returned. The upper affusion was daily performed with great regularity. The nose-bleeding did not return, and in about six weeks the patient was restored to health, although nearly half a year elapsed before she regained her full strength. Disturbance of the system, in consequence of the approaching menses, had apparently produced this attack.

Bloody Flux.

A married man came and related as follows: "My wife has long suffered from bloody flux, and is dying; by the time I reach home she may already be dead. No doctor's help can avail any more. Is there nothing to be done?"

The advice I gave was this: Every quarter of an hour from two to three table-spoonfuls of shave-grass tea, later on two spoonfuls daily will suffice. Upon the body lay a cloth which has been dipped in water half and half with vinegar. Renew this each twenty minutes, and let it remain for two hours.

The bleeding soon stopped, and after two more applications, each of half an hour only, no more were required.

To replace the waste of blood, two table-spoonfuls of milk every hour in addition to her usual diet had the best results. In four weeks the woman was able to resume all her household duties.

I must, however, expressly observe that such means are only to be employed when no doctor can be procured.

Boils.

Inflammation may form outside the body as well as inside, and almost every boil or tumour is attended by some degree of inflammation. When a house is on fire the neighbours all run to the spot, and when a little place on the body burns, the adjacent parts cannot remain indifferent. If, for instance, a small part of the toe be inflamed, no larger than a grain of barley, not only the whole toe will suffer, but even the leg will be affected.

Anna has a dreadful pain in the thumb, although there is not much to be seen. This finger is only slightly swollen and somewhat redder than its companions, yet the pain reaches up to the shoulder-blade. Thinking to cure it, she tightly bandages up the finger, which, however, only increases the evil. The hand and arm swell up, and the whole body is affected.

How, then, should the girl have proceeded to cure the finger? Should she have held it under a pump of cold water in order to cool it and extinguish the heat? Certainly not; the object here not being so much to cool the heat, as to dissolve and secrete the poisonous saps which have occasioned it.

Finger and hand should be swaddled in a cloth dipped in cold water, which must be renewed as often as it absorbs the heat. The finger will probably suppurate and break open, but the boil will never attain such dimensions as it would otherwise have done.

Should there be a sense of oppression and discomfort throughout the body, the Spanish mantle will be of good service.

Bone, Caries of the.

A gentleman of position has a sore toe; he thought that the nail had been injured, and gave the matter no further consideration. Inflammation of the toe set in, and he had recourse to a doctor, who treated him for several weeks, despite which the swelling increased till the whole foot was affected, and walking or standing rendered impossible. The patient himself had no notion of his condition till one day two small bone-splinters detached themselves from the toe.

This aroused his suspicions, not only of his foot, but of all those who had treated it. He sent for me. Caries of the bone had already set in. I caused shave-grass to be boiled, and wrapped the affected foot, as far as the inflammation reached, in cloths dipped in this infusion. The swelling was speedily reduced, the evil arrested, and the patient was soon able to use his foot as before.

About a year later the same disease recurred, but this time on the big toe of the other foot. The doctor made incisions in the toe and employed violent remedies, with the result that the toe was soon healed, although it remained considerably larger and redder than before. Simultaneously, however, the pain in the first foot began to reappear, and after a time the original disease broke out again in its former place.

The mistake made here was that the evil had only been suppressed, not cured, and was therefore sure to reappear again sooner or later. The proper course would have been to treat both feet simultaneously by means of wrappings dipped in shave-grass or oat-straw infusion, which should have been daily applied several times, until there remained no trace of pain or redness on either foot.

Bowels, Complaint of the.

A priest, forty-five years old, relates: "For above twenty-five years I suffered from constipation, and several years ago I went through a course of cold-water cure, which improved my digestion, while leaving the constipation unaltered. In 1885 was added to this a disease of the kidneys, with gravel and complications of the urine. My doctor prescribed a grape cure, followed by a ten days' course of Glauber's salts, which, however, had only the result of leaving behind it a violent catarrh of the bowels. After having tried every possible remedy, I was told that my state was incurable and might be palliated, but never entirely removed. I suffered from sleeplessness, want of appetite, weariness, distaste of work, pain and pressure on the kidneys, constipation, and distension of the lower body. My feet were always cold, my head hot, the rest of my body inclined to profuse perspiration. In this condition I resolved once more to have recourse to cold water, which I had previously been warned against."

The following applications were prescribed to this gentleman: Daily one upper affusion, one back affusion, one sitz-bath—to which were subsequently added, according to expediency, a semi-bath, knee affusion, and water-walking. The best results were, however, achieved by the Spanish mantle, for which he conceived a warm friendship. After twelve weeks' treatment, the digestion was completely restored, and the body gained 13 lb. in weight.

Bowels, Inflammation of the.

An overseer relates: "For years I have had violent, sometimes almost unbearable, pains and cramps in the bowels. For long I have not been able to eat without great pain, succeeded invariably by diarrhœa. I have tried many remedies, all without avail."

The appearance of this man, who stood in the prime of life, was very sickly. His eyes were dull, the complexion pale, and the figure emaciated. How was he to be cured?

Each week he took—

1. Three sitz-baths.

2. Every morning and evening the breast and under body were washed in water mixed with vinegar.

In four weeks the man was released from his sufferings. As internal remedy, he merely took twelve drops of wormwood twice daily in warm water.

Brain, Inflammation of the.

Wherever inflammation arises, the blood has a tendency to flow to that part and concentrate itself there. In cases of inflammation of the brain, it is therefore of great importance to draw down the blood from the head to the extremities, as well as to reduce the heat at the affected spot. The applications to be used are as follows:—

The feet up to the knee should be swaddled in cloths dipped in vinegar and water, and the arms swaddled in like fashion up to the elbow. Should the feet be very cold, then the cloth may at first be dipped in hot water. Both swaddlings to be renewed every hour or half-hour, according to the degree of heat absorbed. These swaddlings may be succeeded by a lower compress. On the head a simple cold-water compress, or else a long wet bandage wound tightly round the neck. Whichever of these is employed must be renewed half-hourly. These means, if properly and consistently applied, will prevent the heat from attaining a high degree, and accelerate recovery. As internal remedies, pure cold water, given in one or two spoonfuls occasionally, will always remain the best; but instead of water, an infusion of *fœnum græcum* may be taken.

Burns.

A peasant's house was burnt down. The peasant received such injuries from the fire on face and hands as to be absolutely unrecognisable. From the fingers and from half the arm skin and flesh hung down in ragged strips. In inexpressible agony the unfortunate man called upon death to release him. The doctor applied several plasters to the wounds, but gave no hope of recovery.

Chance brought me to the bedside of the patient. I could not bear to witness this suffering, and tried to think of some means of relieving his pain, so as at least to enable him to die quietly. I caused all the stiff adhesive plasters to be removed, and forming a paste out of sour cream, linseed-oil, and white of egg, I painted this over the raw wounds, so as to protect them from the outer air, covering each spot carefully with a soft linen rag, which adhered closely to the flesh, and above the rags I placed another dry linen cloth. At intervals of two hours I removed the outer cloth, and remoistened the lower rag with the same mixture. Twice daily the lower rags were likewise removed and replaced by fresh ones. In an incredibly short time the man was cured. As internal remedies I gave him twice daily one spoonful of olive-oil.

Under this air-tight covering the new skin was quickly formed, and the rigid attention to cleanliness prevented the wounds from suppurating. In fourteen days the man was almost well again.

For slighter burns or scalds, pickled cabbage (Sauer-kraut) or potato-scrapings may be employed with good results.

CANCER.

This is a very common disease nowadays. There is hardly a part of the body which may not be destroyed by cancer or cancerous complaints. If the disease be far advanced, then I do not dare to apply water; blood and saps are already corrupted.

Cancer is sometimes infectious, especially if there be a predisposition to decomposition of blood and saps in an individual.

I knew a married couple who went to visit a cousin afflicted with cancer of the tongue. Without at all understanding the nature of this dreadful complaint, they were both alarmed on seeing the ravages produced. The woman's tongue began to swell up within four days, and the man's under lip got inflamed and sore. "We have caught the disease," they came lamenting to me. I endeavoured to calm the terrified persons, but without success. I advised them to wash out the whole mouth, and particularly the affected spot, four times daily with alum-water, and on the following day to repeat the process with water of aloe; likewise every second day to take a head vapour bath, alternated with a throat-swathing.

The two persons were completely cured of their complaints. I myself would never have believed it possible that mere fright could convey this terrible disease. I was told later that a doctor had pronounced the people to have been infected by the illness.

I have successfully cured many cases of cancer in early stages. All applications were chiefly directed towards purifying the blood and saps.

Catarrh or Cold.

Most catarrhs are produced by coming quickly out of the cold air—perhaps perspiring—into a heated room. Exposure to cold draught may likewise be the cause. Usually a sense of pressure and contraction is felt at once in chest, throat, or nose. There is a feeling as of a little round ball in the throat. If we disregard these first symptoms of a beginning catarrh, it strikes root and spreads itself out. Those who are used to much warm clothing, and whose organs are consequently enervated, are most easily attacked. It would be easy to keep all colds at a distance were we to harden our bodies by proper means.

What must we do in order to remain free of colds? An example will tell us. I have been walking rapidly for an hour in cold weather: the thermometer marks 5° F. Without transition I come into a room whose temperature is 64° F. This rapid change of 59° cannot be accomplished with impunity, it must bring danger. It would have been wiser if I had walked more slowly for the last five to twenty minutes, and then had paused a little in the passage (always in motion) before entering the room. In this manner the heightened temperature would have had time to cool somewhat, and the perspiration to disperse.

If you feel the consequences of your imprudence, if you are conscious of a little lump in the throat, go out once more into the open air and take exercise for half an hour. This will effectively remove and dissolve all superfluous matter in the throat.

Hoarseness is nothing but the communication of catarrh to the speaking organs. A silver bell produces no tone if it be muffled; and the most splendid voice encumbered by inflammation will give no sound. Remove the catarrh, and its companion hoarseness will speedily follow.

CHOLERA.

How much dreaded is cholera! In order to ensure ourselves against floods we regulate the rivers and build up dams; and when a forest burns we dig ditches to prevent the flames from spreading. Water fulfils the same office with regard to cholera. It averts the danger, and surrounds us, so to say, with a dam or ditch.

The universal rule applying to cholera is, that whoever can be made to perspire freely is saved, but that he who cannot do so is lost.

Once at night I was summoned to a poor maid-servant. Twenty times she had already vomited, and twenty times had suffered from violent purging. The doctor was two hours distant. The girl wished to be prepared for death, feeling convinced that this dreadful illness must prove fatal. Hands and feet were like lumps of ice, the face pale, the features drawn and pinched; all the signs of approaching dissolution were there. I instantly sought to produce sweating, as in my opinion everything depended upon this—life or death. The housewife brought two large coarse linen sheets. I dipped these in hot water, and applied them hot, folded together on chest and abdomen. Beneath the sheets and against the bare skin I had previously placed a single cloth dipped in vinegar. The wet hot compress was covered over and secured against the air by a feather quilt as warm and heavy as the patient could endure. Rapidly heat penetrated into the diseased body, and in fifteen minutes the whole frame was warmed throughout. Twenty minutes more, and large drops of perspiration appeared on the face. I caused the linen sheets to be redipped in hot water. Soon the cramps entirely ceased, and with them the retching and vomiting. In order to promote the internal heat, the patient was made to drink a cupful of fennel tea boiled in milk (one spoonful of ground fennel boiled in milk three minutes), and taken as hot as possible. The sick girl fell into profuse perspiration, and was saved.

The treatment of convalescents from cholera, though simple, is important, and should never be neglected. They should daily apply a lower compress for one hour; likewise daily an upper compress for the same length of time. My patient did this for ten to twelve days, and was completely cured. A second case was treated in the same manner and with the same result.

I cannot refrain from two further remarks.

When the first symptoms of cholera appear, as vomiting, violent purging, cramps, &c., the patient should at once be put to bed. Country people are often too hard against themselves in this respect, and act unwisely in resisting the illness. Internally there should be given some warm beverage to drink. If cramps are threatening, or if the feet be cold, a warm compress should be laid on the body, not longer than for three-quarters of an hour. Likewise, and for the same length of time, a warm lower compress. If heat and perspiration be created, then the game is won.

Care as to diet must be observed until the system has completely regained its former regularity. Of the customary food the lighter dishes should be selected. As beverage, give preference to warm milk, which is medicine and nourishment combined.

If the cholera is raging in a place, then trust to God and be fearless! As precautionary measures, daily wash the chest and lower body morn and evening, and chew ten to twelve juniper-berries. In default of these, peppercorns may be used. For 4d. you can buy a great many of these. Five peppercorns taken twice a-day will warm the stomach, assist digestion, and dispel unwholesome gases.

Cholerine.

In most places some cases of cholerine occur every year, and I myself have had many such patients. Cholerine is a small edition of cholera, a very unwelcome, though far less dreaded visitor. Vomiting, violent purging, sometimes cramps, more or less severe, follow in its train.

My applications for cholerine are identical with those for cholera, modified as to number and strength according to the greater or lesser violence of the complaint. Forty patients, simultaneously attacked by cholerine, were all thus treated with complete success.

Colic.

Colic, with purging or with vomiting, sometimes appears suddenly, apparently without cause. It may have been occasioned by catching cold, overheating, or by some unwholesome food or drink. The patient should at once be put to bed, and warmly, though not oppressively, covered up. A hot bottle may be placed on the abdomen (poor people often make use of a piece of heated brick for the purpose). As an internal remedy make him drink a pint of milk in which fennel or caraway has been boiled. This simple household medicine will suffice.

With regard to diet, so long as the condition is unchanged, the food must be of the very simplest and lightest; salt, pepper, and all such condiments are to be avoided. As beverage, pure water or milk, or at the utmost a little wine and water.

Congestions.

An official thus complained: "I suffer from difficulty in breathing, cramps in the throat, and violent headache. Sometimes I lie awake all night on account of the congestions and pain in the head. For years I have not been able to go to stool without the assistance of medicine. Moreover, I have cramps in the chest, and when these descend to the abdomen, I suffer great pain. I cannot protect myself from cold; hands and feet are invariably cold. My position in life would be a pleasant one were I not so continually tormented by suffering. I have been to various watering-places, but have found no help. My former stoutness has given way to emaciation. If water brings me no help," he said plaintively, "then I am lost."

The treatment was as follows:—

1. Walking in wet grass daily, morning and evening, for a considerable time, which relieved him exceedingly and diverted the headache.
2. Twice weekly a short swathing.
3. Once a-week a Spanish mantle.

In order to promote stools, during several days a table-spoonful of water to be swallowed every half-hour; and in case of greater inconvenience, a piece of aloe as large as a pea, with half a spoonful of sugar dissolved in hot water, and likewise taken in spoonfuls half-hourly.

CONSTIPATION.

Many persons suffer from diarrhœa, but a yet greater number are afflicted with constipation. These sufferers have mostly recourse to artificial means, which, though fulfilling the immediate object of promoting stools, have always in the long-run a detrimental effect on the system.

Something is usually wrong with the general health of those who suffer from constipation. One of the first questions which every doctor addresses to a patient is regarding the regularity and nature of his stools. If these be in order, then the first conditions of health are there; but in the reverse case it may be confidently assumed that disease has set in, which, if the cause be not removed, may lead to severe illness, or even to premature death.

Constipated subjects should take every morning, from breakfast-time till noon, one table-spoonful of water every half-hour. These small doses will achieve greater results than water imbibed in large quantities. In the afternoon the patient may likewise take a spoonful of water every half-hour or every hour. This frequent but sparse irrigation is of soothing effect, and increases the saps. The patient may however drink, notwithstanding, whenever he is thirsty.

Instead of water a great many different sorts of tea, prepared from familiar plants, may be employed. Who does not know the sloe-blossom? Its tea is of excellent effect. Elder-flower tea cools, dissolves, and removes internal heat; mixed with three to four grains of aloe it acts as a gentle cooling laxative: six to eight elder-leaves, plucked in spring-time and made into tea, are likewise of cooling effect. Half a cupful morning and evening is the proper dose.

Cold-water applications are to be used in conjunction with these internal remedies. Let the patient wash over the abdomen vigorously with a handful of water morning or evening. This practice, though simple, is very effective in removing constipation, and will be sufficient for weakly persons.

Those who require something stronger may take a cold knee affusion from time to time, of one to three minutes' duration; and if this likewise prove too weak, and should the patient suffer from much internal heat, a lower compress may be taken twice weekly. The upper compress will likewise do good service; or else a cold sitz-bath twice or thrice weekly. A cold full bath, if taken rapidly, is also not to be despised.

All the afore-mentioned applications will serve to rouse the indolent system and incite it to renewed activity. The wheels being freshly oiled, the whole machine runs smoothly again, and healthly evacuations will not fail to set in.

Nothing can surpass the effect of water; and what is easier than to drink water and to wash with it?

Consumption.

Like a serpent in the grass lying in ambush for its prey, so consumption often lurks in the system long before its presence is suspected. Its origin is a decomposition, which sets in at some particular spot, whence it spreads throughout the body, destroying certain organs. This may take place in the chest, lungs, pleura, abdomen, intestines, kidneys, throat, windpipe, &c. Wherever this corruption takes place, there follow disorders of the circulation and secretions. The person thus afflicted is like a blighted tree, whose leaves begin to wither and fall off; neither sunshine nor fresh air can restore it. The same may be said of a consumptive person. His blood, his secretions decline, and he goes out like a rushlight, unable to live.

When consumption has once struck root and corrupted an internal organ, then the patient is doomed. When, however, the disease has but slightly attacked some part, then, by means of water, a cure may easily be affected. It is a melancholy fact that the first symptons of the disease are so easily overlooked and disregarded. The patient has a slight painless cough, with little or no expectoration. If sometimes the cough increases, the patient consoles himself by the reflection that it is only a slight catarrh, which will soon be dispelled. Even when the body begins to fall off, and strength to decline, he is seldom seriously alarmed. The catarrh has lasted longer this time, he thinks; but he is still able to fulfil the duties of his profession. Such patients have usually suffered more than they are aware off at this stage of their illness: the formation of blood has decreased, the secretions have lessened, the affected spots spread ever further. If the patient then seeks assistance, it is mostly too late, and what he does and employs often only serves to shorten his span of life. I mention this as a warning not to neglect any catarrhal complaints, of whatsoever kind or description. Where consumption is far advanced, water should never be applied, nature being no longer sufficiently vigorous to engage in a tussle with the cold element. This were as foolish as if a weak puny youth were to attempt to wrestle with an athlete. An advanced stage of consumption is recognised by the patient's frequent cough, accompanied by much expectoration; by his difficult breathing and impaired appetite, &c. So long as the expectorated matter floats on the water's surface, there is yet room for hope. If it sinks, then all help is mostly in vain; let the patient resign himself to God's holy will, and calmly prepare for death.

Beginning consumption may, however, be often arrested by means of cold water, as I can testify by many examples. Cold water serves to revive and invigorate the withered body, and acts like oil on the wheel of a rusty machine: it promotes a healthy circulation, and infuses new life into the system, dissolving and withdrawing unhealthy secretions, as a winnowing machine removes the chaff. Care must be taken, however, never to make use of too violent applications, which would but serve to aggravate the complaint.

Should the disease have its seat in the upper part of the body, then the upper affusion is an excellent application, combined with the knee affusion, the latter for half a minute only. In favourable weather, walking barefoot in wet grass is not to be surpassed in its effects. This will strengthen the body, and no one need fear to harm themselves by this practice. Walking on wet stones is also good.

A word here as to diet for these patients, into whose ears is mostly dinned the axiom, "Eat and drink well." The simplest diet is the best; nothing heating, spiced, or sour should be taken. I have frequently had occasion to make the singular observation that consumptive persons have a violent and unnatural craving for everything salt and sour: this symptom alone has often helped me to detect the illness. Above all, milk may be recommended as nourishment, but should only be taken in combination with other food, for fear of its causing aversion to the patient. Also, strengthening soups are much to be recommended, but always alternated with other nourishment. Light simple puddings and farinaceous preparations, free from all artifice, may also be taken. Water always remains the best beverage, sometimes mixed with a little wine. Curdled sour milk is likewise wholesome. I do not recommend either beer or wine.

A last remark may here find place. In the more advanced stages of this complaint, violent fever sometimes appears, combined with perspiration and shivering fits. These cannot be completely removed; but some relief may be afforded to the patient if he daily wash over vigorously his chest, back, and lower body with fresh water.

An excellent school teacher had been treated by a celebrated doctor for some time, without result. Not being able longer to perform her duties, she was pensioned provisionally for three-quarters of a year. As at the end of this time her condition had nowise improved, the doctor in his certificate pronounced her to be incurable, and consequently unfit to resume her profession. Some friends having advised her to try cold water, she took a lodging in the neighbourhood of my parish. At first she was so weak that she could scarcely walk for half an hour. She went through a course of cold-water applications according to directions, and was completely cured in from four to five weeks. She then desired to be reinstated in her situation as teacher, but had considerable trouble in obtaining this, for no one would believe in the fact of her cure. She went in person to the minister, who was surprised at her blooming appearance, no less than at the definition "incurable" on her certificate. It is now six years since she resumed her duties, and has been in uninterrupted enjoyment of perfect health. I do not know what complaint the doctor had found in this patient, and never ascertained whether it was supposed to be decline or consumption; all symptoms, however, pointed towards consumption. The young lady had already lost a brother, whose condition had been precisely identical with her own.

It was high time, but yet still time, to arrest the disease; this was done by cold water. The remedies employed were: Much open air, frequent walking barefoot in wet grass, baths from the slightest and weakest applications up to the last and strongest, all taken cold. To these were added herb teas, and a simple nourishing country diet.

A man came and related: "There is something wrong with my chest and throat. I used to have a violent catarrh, then I lost my voice almost completely, and for weeks I suffered from an intense burning in throat and chest, accompanied by fever. I have had several doctors, and was treated with various inhalations. I sometimes obtained slight relief, but no real help. I am now quite emaciated, and can no longer do anything but walk about a little. My feet are always cold, my appetite better than formerly."

The applications were—

1. Twice daily a knee affusion or walking in water.
2. Morning and afternoon daily an upper affusion.
3. Two little cupfuls of fenugreek tea twice daily.
4. Every second day a cold sitz-bath for the space of one minute.

This course to be continued for three weeks.

Cramps.

I was called to a sick person who was trembling in the whole body, and who threw herself about in bed from side to side. The patient herself was unable to speak, but her mother related:

"My daughter suffers from terrible headaches, great oppression on chest and stomach; hands and feet are always icy cold, and wet with a clammy perspiration. She has been married for three-quarters of a year: for ten weeks she was in good health, then these symptoms began, slightly at first, but always increasing till they reached this point. She can eat nothing but a few spoonfuls of clear soup or coffee; everything which doctors have given her, and the injections administered in order to produce artificial sleep, have but aggravated her condition."

I gave the following advice to the patient:

Twice daily to put the feet in water reaching above the calves, and simultaneously to wash over the feet with a sponge or towel; immediately after to hold the arms in water up to the shoulder for one minute, and wash over the hands; hands and feet to be then covered up with the warm bedclothes; every morning and afternoon the patient was to take twelve drops of camomile extract in from six to eight spoonfuls of hot water. As nourishment, three or four spoonfuls of milk or of malt coffee were to be administered from time to time; or, best of all, milk and malt coffee taken in alternate portions.

In twelve days this person was so far restored that the appetite for habitual simple nourishment had returned: the cramps had vanished, the oppressive pains in chest and stomach had ceased, likewise the headache; hands and feet were warm.

As further applications, she continued to stand daily in cold water as above, twice weekly a warm foot-bath with salt and ashes for fourteen minutes, and once in the week a complete lavation from bed. Instead of camomile she now took wormwood and sage, ten to twelve drops in warm water. The patient recovered so far as to be able to go again to church, and to resume her household work; and in order completely to regain her strength she only required to take a cold lavation, or, better still, a semi-bath twice in the week.

Croup.

A father came to me lamenting that his four-year-old daughter had croup. "The child," he said, "has got it just like the three other children who all died. They all died very quickly, and so will this child. It can hardly breathe or cough. Head and body are much inflated. What shall I do? It would require four hours to fetch the doctor, and by that time the child will be dead."

The answer was: "Good father, go home, heat some

water with vinegar, dip a towel in it, wring it out, and wrap it round the child's neck. Over this put a dry cloth, and let this swathing remain on three-quarters of an hour. Then dip the towel anew in vinegar-and-water. Continue to do this for six hours, always renewing at the end of three-quarters of an hour. After six hours remove the throat compress and cover the neck lightly, then apply to the child with the same towel, dipped afresh in vinegar and water, a short swathing with a dry cloth over it, covering up the child carefully but not too heavily. Let the little one lie quiet for one hour. After one hour remove the coverings, and let the child remain in bed covered up as usual. If after from six to eight hours the cough and difficulty in breathing are still present, then repeat the throat compress as before. You will soon experience its good effects."

The father followed my directions, and after thirty hours the child, whom he had already believed to be lost, had regained its usual health and spirits.

The same cure might have been effected with cold water and vinegar, in place of warm, and renewed as above every three-quarters of an hour. When the heat proves obstinate, the feet and legs may also be swathed in wet bandages to above the calves.

Debilitation.

A smith, forty-six years old, came and complained: "My hands have so decreased in strength during the last two years that I can hardly wield the hammer. Not only have I lost two-thirds of my strength, but my hands have dwindled to half their former size; otherwise my health is tolerably good, except that for half a year my legs have been weaker, and often pain me towards evening. I also frequently feel a sense of pressure on the upper back."

On the emaciated hands the veins are hardly perceptible: it is easy to see that the hands are receiving no nourishment—hence the weakness, stiffness, and sensation of cold. Agglomeration of blood in the neck and its neighbourhood may be the cause why the blood does not circulate to all parts of the body.

For fourteen days the smith held his arms for half an hour daily in a hay-flower bath, and once daily, at another time of day, for two minutes in cold water; to this was added a shawl thrice weekly. Already, during the cure, the arms grew stronger, the veins were refilled, the agglomerations were dissolved. After a fortnight, a daily upper and lower affusion was taken, twice a-week a warm hay-flower bath, and twice a cold-water arm-bath. The man persevered in these applications, and was able to resume the exercise of his trade. As internal remedies, he daily took twenty drops of wormwood extract in warm water.

DECLINE.

We frequently see persons who have rapidly grown stout. This is usually dreaded, because experience has shown that such individuals are not long-lived. In the same way we meet many in whom a contrary process has taken place, and whose strength shows a rapid decrease. These are like the grass on the field, which to-day is green and to-morrow withered; and what is strangest in the complaint is, that persons thus attacked are often unconscious of any serious indisposition. They mostly complain of weariness, low spirits, and either excessive or deficient appetite. If assistance be not at hand, these semi-withered plants will rapidly fade away; like a feeble rushlight, they will soon be extinguished. Decline is thereby distinguished from consumption, that whereas in the latter the disease invariably proceeds from some particular organ, as lungs, chest, larynx, &c., whence it spreads throughout the body, the former more resembles a general dissolution of the system, in which we vainly seek to discover a tangible reason for the complaint.

A tolerably stout gentleman rejoiced in good health. Habits and diets were carefully regulated. Of a sudden he noticed that his strength and corpulence began to decrease. He grew subject to fits of giddiness, and often could scarcely stand alone. Within six weeks he had lost 72 lb. in weight. The large and singularly handsome man of a little while ago now wavered and tottered like a broken reed, lifeless and withered as a blighted forest-tree. All medical remedies were in vain: the patient looked forward to his approaching end with painful certitude.

In this state of mind and body he came to me: I did not recognise him, although he had been a former acquaintance. I greatly doubted the possibility of recovery, but advised him, nevertheless, to make a last attempt with cold water.

Declining nature required to be braced and fortified, and the suicidal process arrested. Two or three times daily the patient walked barefoot in wet grass or on wet stones. Every other day he took an upper and lower compress, once in the week a Spanish mantle. These applications were followed by a semi-bath weekly, one short swathing, and an upper and lower compress.

The semi-baths were then exchanged for whole baths, of which two different sorts were taken—viz., cold baths of one minute, and warm ones repeated twice over, each time with transition into cold water —of each kind one in the week; likewise once a-week a complete lavation. As a final cure, and to ward off a relapse, I prescribed weekly a whole bath, an upper affusion with knee affusion, and occasionally a Spanish mantle. The patient's daily portion of beer was reduced from four or five glasses to two glasses, and the diet was ordered to be simple and nourishing.

By the end of the first week improvement was already visible. After eight weeks the convalescent was able to resume his daily occupations and duties. As his strength so also his bodily weight increased, and he is to-day still a strong, healthy, and handsome man.

Delirium Tremens.

A man, thirty-six years old, had drunk much beer, eaten little, and during a considerable time had nourished himself almost exclusively on beer. *Delirium tremens* had already set in, and was so far advanced as to be generally observable. He was also afflicted with rheumatic pains, cramps, and occasional headaches. Though drunkenness is very difficult to cure, yet this patient had the firm desire to be rid of his wretched complaint, no matter at what sacrifice.

This man was completely cured within three weeks by means of the following applications:—

First day.—(*a*) Upper affusion and knee affusion.

(*b*) Water-standing, water-walking, and holding the arms in water.

Second day.—(*a*) Semi-bath. (*b*) Upper affusion with knee affusion.

Third day.—(*a*) Sitz-bath. (*b*) Upper affusion.

Fourth day.—(*a*) Semi-bath. (*b*) Whole bath.

This was continued until the cure was complete: all unhealthy symptoms disappeared, the appearance improved, appetite returned, and the craving for strong drink completely disappeared. It must specially be remarked that during the cure there appeared eruptions on various parts of the body, by means of which the poisonous matter was thrown off.

Diarrhœa.

Some people are subject to occasional apparently causeless attacks of severe diarrhœa. These attacks are sometimes regular—that is to say, they invariably recur once or twice a-year—sometimes, however, they are of quite irregular appearance. Persons thus visited usually feel quite well both before and after the attack. The regular recurring diarrhœa denotes that the patient's vigorous nature elects this manner of throwing off accumulations of superfluous matter.

Against such diarrhœas I have nothing to prescribe: on the contrary, I warn every one against trying to arrest the laxation, which, evidently dictated by nature, is of most frequent occurrence in spring and autumn.

The matter stands differently with regard to irregular diarrhœas: these, often attended by pain, are a sign of the presence of unhealthy matter in the system, which if not removed will prove pernicious. In such cases some internal organ is assuredly affected, and if the complaint be not seen to in time, the patient is not likely to reach old age. Diarrhœa is likewise often the precursor of serious illness. In treating a convalescent, it is of the first importance to act upon the abdomen: these applications, however, must be varied and alternated by others directed to the whole body. Violent diarrhœa should never be averted suddenly; the unhealthy matter must be removed by degrees, and the internal organs fortified in such manner as to enable nature to reject all further intrusion of superfluous matter or to expel it at proper times.

As internal remedies, tea of wormwood and sage, or of milfoil and centaury, one to two cupfuls daily, or else daily swallow from six to ten juniper-berries. Any of the aforementioned will render good service, and will tend to strengthen the digestion again.

Should the diarrhœa prove violent and obstinate, half a spoonful of juniper extract may be taken twice daily in warm water.

As external applications a compress on the abdomen, dipped in vinegar-and-water, or else in a pine-tree decoction, three or four times weekly during an hour and a half, and a short swathing once a-week, will suffice for the first fortnight. After that, in order to strengthen the system, one or two semi-baths, followed by a lavation of the upper body, may be taken every week. Likewise weekly, one or two complete lavations, applied at night straight away from the warm bed. This second course of treatment to be continued for four weeks. If, later on, the patient will still continue to take at least one semi-bath or complete lavation every week, the whole system will be thereby so consolidated and strengthened, as completely to banish the original complaint, unless it has its root in some deep-seated organic disease.

Diphtheria.

Those attacked by this disease should strive—

1. To dissolve and remove the accumulated unhealthy matter as rapidly as possible.
2. To act upon the whole system in such manner that the disturbed circulation, which is the surest barometer of fever, should be restored to its normal condition.

Let the patient first take a vapour head-bath, and some twenty to twenty-four minutes later a lavation. After six to eight hours the wet shawl may be applied for one and a half hour, to be renewed however—that is, redipped in fresh water—at the end of each half-hour. After this, let the patient take a vapour foot-bath, to be immediately followed by a cold semi-bath accompanied by lavation of the upper body. This last proceeding—bath and lavation together—should not occupy more than one minute. Then again the shawl for one and a half hour as above. When this course of treatment has been gone through, begin again in the same order as here mentioned, but in such manner that one application only takes place in each half-day. Gargling with shave-grass infusion will likewise assist the process, and should be practised from four to five times daily. This noxious disease will soon yield to these remedies.

Should the patient fall into a quiet sleep, he should on no account be disturbed, even for the sake of an application. Sleep is the surest sign that nature is beginning to settle down to quiet and order, and its invigorating effects will assist the cold-water action by-and-by.

This rule likewise holds good for cases in which the patient falls asleep during an application (swathing, compress, &c.) Do not disturb him. When the application has done its work he will awake spontaneously.

A father came to me and related: "My child, aged eleven, can no longer swallow, and has hardly been able to breathe for three days. He is burning hot and delirious. I wrapped a wet cloth round his neck, but it has done no good. What shall I do to save the child from choking?"

The unhappy father's grief, and still more the failure of the cold-water swathing, determined me to accompany him to his son's bedside. There lay the child, a picture of woe, and to all appearance doomed, for there were signs which seemed to exclude all hope. Let us try, however, in God's name!

Every half-hour during a whole day the back, chest, and lower body were well washed over, and as the fearful heat still continued, a cloth dipped in water was laid on the belly as sole covering. This must subdue the heat. Next day the father came and related: "The child is already able to swallow a little; but the cheeks on both sides are beginning to swell up towards the jawbones. His speech is hardly intelligible, but I am happy beyond measure that he is now able to speak at all." The father was told to apply compresses dipped in vinegar-and-water to the swollen cheeks, and to renew these every half-hour. At the same time he was to go on washing the child on back, chest, and belly, as above directed, as often as heat and uneasiness were felt.

A gargle made of one tea-spoonful of fenugreek boiled in half a pint of water, frequently administered in spoonfuls, had an excellent effect. Tea of mallow, great mullein, or milfoil might likewise have been employed. It is also good to swallow daily three to four tea-spoonfuls of salad-oil. This rapidly dispels the internal heat.

The child was saved, and is still to-day in excellent health.

Dizziness.

A priest in the prime of life suffered from a gradual and perceptible decrease of strength, especially in the legs. Only with great effort was he able to walk a quarter of an hour, and had the sensation as though his legs were about to give way under him. Besides this complaint he suffered so much from dizziness that he could not stand in an open space without holding on by some fixed object. When he had to turn round at the altar, he was always obliged to steady himself. Whenever the dizziness decreased, he felt a violent oppression on the chest, and a sense of anxiety as if a paralytic stroke were imminent.

The patient had taken much mineral water and medicine, but without result. His appearance did not betoken suffering, and the appetite was good, but the sleep much impaired.

Treatment: Having suspended the duties of his vocation for three weeks, he daily walked barefoot (in grass, water up to the knee, or on wet stones), received daily two upper affusions and a knee affusion, later on semi-baths and full baths, taken while in a state of complete perspiration. At the conclusion of his cure the patient made the attempt to walk four hours in one day, which was accomplished without fatigue. He now felt quite healthy, and happy to resume his sacerdotal duties.

A gentleman, aged seventy-four, related: "I suffer frequently from violent dizziness, and have at times a heavy pressure on the head; my feet are often cold, and when my head is free, I regularly experience great discomfort in the abdomen. I never can go to stool without artificial assistance. The book, 'My Water Cure,' has caused me to ask whether at my advanced age cold water may still be employed with success? If such be the case, then I will go into cold water as readily as the youngest; but if not, then I shall calmly resign myself to my fate."

In three weeks' time the old gentleman felt so well that he regretted having made over his duties to another.

The applications here used consisted in the following:—

First day.—In the morning, complete lavation of the upper body with vinegar-and-water, followed by a knee affusion; in the evening, a warm foot-bath, with salt and ashes, for fourteen minutes.

Second day.—In the morning, upper affusion of the contents of one watering-can, immediately succeeded by walking on wet stones (for five minutes); afternoon, a cold sitz-bath for one minute.

Third day.—Walking in water in the morning for two minutes, directly after this holding the arms in water; afternoon, an upper affusion; towards evening, a sitz-bath.

Fourth day.—In the morning, walking for three minutes in water reaching to the knees, directly followed by holding the arms in water for two minutes; afternoon, a back affusion.

Fifth day.—Back affusion in the morning; in the afternoon, a semi-bath.

In this manner the latter strongest applications were pursued. The dizziness completely disappeared, the digestion became regular, unwholesome gases were expelled, the normal temperature was re-established, and the whole machine restored to order. The old man regained an almost juvenile freshness and the most cheerful humour.

Some readers may be surprised that in this case, and in view of the patient's advanced age, but one single warm application was employed. The reason was simply that the old man still possessed sufficient strength and latent heat to endure the action of cold water, which, when practicable, is always of far greater effect than any warm course of treatment.

Dropsy.

After continuous rain, where the soil is not porous and there is little sunshine, the water is apt to form into pools and marshes, which, becoming stagnant and foul, are of pernicious influence on the plants which grow in their neighbourhood.

In much the same manner is dropsy formed, which is mostly developed in the systems of those whose blood and secretions are of watery composition. Every organ, every part of the body, draws its life and nourishment from the blood. From unhealthy blood, as from a foul stagnant marsh, neither strength nor life can be drawn—hence the flaccid loose flesh, withered vessels, and agglomerations, all foreboding symptoms of dropsy.

Even by the appearance of such patients it is easy to detect the complaint. Young people suddenly age, the complexion becomes dull, nerves and muscles hang loosely on the bones, like the cords of an unstrung instrument; in various places, especially about the eyes, little water-bags begin to form.

There are various kinds of dropsy. If these water-bags are formed between flesh and skin, then we have dropsy of the skin. If in the cavity of the abdomen the water assembles in large pools, then it is called dropsy of the belly. There is also dropsy of the head, heart, chest, &c. Dropsy is often the consequence of recent severe illness, and is apt to appear particularly after scarlet fever, when the poisonous matter has been imperfectly expelled.

When dropsy has spread throughout the body and attained large dimensions, then it is mostly incurable because of the lack of blood. In the early stages, and before decomposition has set in, it is often readily cured, so to say, by pumping out the stagnant water. Some examples will illustrate my meaning.

The body of a peasant-woman, aged about forty-eight, began to swell up in such a manner that she could hardly walk. Her weakness was very great, and she breathed with difficulty. I advised her to express rosemary in wine, and daily to drink two wine-glassfuls of this rosemary wine (about half a pint). The wine greatly strengthened the patient, and expelled much water. Furthermore, she daily took a short swathing of an hour and a half for several days, and during four weeks two semi-baths daily of one minute, combined with lavation of the upper body. The peasant-woman recovered completely, and was able to resume all the duties of her state of life.

A boy aged twelve had apparently recovered from scarlet fever. After six weeks he got dropsy, and the whole body swelled up. A shirt dipped in salt water and applied three days in succession for one and a half hour restored the boy to perfect health.

A woman aged fifty-four was attacked by dropsy of the belly. The legs and body were, as I was informed, terribly swollen. The patient's daughter was told to prepare daily for her mother some danewort tea (two pinches of danewort boiled in half a pint of water for three minutes), to be drunk in two or three doses. Besides this, she daily received a lower swathing of one hour during eight days. During the following ten days the swathing was only applied every second day, and during the last fortnight every third day. The patient completely recovered in three weeks' time, large quantities of water being secreted through the urine.

Danewort root has always rendered me the best services in cases of dropsy of the belly, while rosemary is most to be recommended for dropsy of the chest and heart.

An excellent outward application for heart dropsy is an upper and lower compress applied daily. As internal medicine, two glasses of rosemary wine should be taken.

I must not forget to remark here that warm water,

in whatever form, should never be used in cases of dropsy. Neither vapour nor warm baths are permissible, because they would but serve to aggravate the disease, by increasing the flaccidity and limpness of nerves and organs which chiefly characterises it. The coldest applications are here always the best: they should not, however, be employed otherwise than in the manner prescribed; when the blood is poor, then the latent heat is likewise small.

Dysentery.

Dysentery is the sister of cholera. There is much similarity between these two complaints. Dysentery usually begins with violent spasms in the abdomen and excessive purging, the stools being mixed with blood.

The quickest way of curing dysentery is to dip a folded linen cloth in hot water and vinegar, and lay it on the body. Of surprising effect as internal medicine is the extract of bilberry, which should be wanting in no household pharmacy. Two tablespoonfuls of this essence, taken in hot water twice daily, is the proper dose. Should the patient's condition not have materially improved by the second day, the compress on the body may be repeated as well as the medicine.

Like a worm, Joseph was writhing in his bed; the cramps sometimes rolled him about like a ball. He screamed aloud with pain. More than a pint of blood had been purged from him. Two spoonfuls of the aforementioned bilberry extract, taken morning and afternoon, restored order in a very short time.

Anna, a woman over fifty years of age, is wailing in fearful cramps. Purging with blood made her fear that she was attacked with cholera. The vinegar compress on the body, and bilberry extract taken internally, cured her within a day. When no bilberries are procurable, then fennel boiled in milk will render good service.

EAR COMPLAINTS.

Who could enumerate the various causes from which disease may proceed, and how often an illness may continue permanently to affect an organ after the original complaint has been removed? The more delicate and noble the organ, the more liable it is to be impaired, and the more difficult its cure. The ear is one of the noblest organs in the human frame, and we may frequently lose our hearing through illness or an irregular mode of life.

A mother came to me and related: "My daughter had scarlet fever, from which she indeed recovered, but since that time she has never been quite well. She complains now of one, now of the other thing, but her greatest affliction is having almost completely lost her hearing. All remedies we tried have been unavailing."

This girl has evidently not been completely cured of her illness, and not only the ears but other parts of the body must likewise be affected. The cure must therefore be directed towards the whole system, not to the ears alone.

The following applications will be the best:—

1. A wet shirt for one and a half hour.

2. A shawl one and a half hour, to be renewed at the end of three-quarters of an hour. Simultaneously with the shawl the legs are each to be bandaged with

wet cloths (dipped in warm water) for the same length of time.

3. A complete lavation taken from bed, with particular care as to washing the ears and back of the head.

4. A bandage dipped in warm water secured over the ears for two hours and renewed at the end of each half hour.

5. A head swathing.

These five applications to be continued for a considerable length of time, at least one application daily.

Of good effect would likewise be once in the week a warm oat-straw bath (95° to 100° F.) for twenty-five minutes, concluded by a cold lavation. These applications will restore order to the system, but the warm bandage over the ears may be continued for some length of time.

Ears, Singing in the.

A person suffered from singing in the ears, weak nerves, trembling in hands and feet, pale complexion and sunken eyes. Various doctors had been consulted. One had declared the complaint to be caused by nerves, a second from a suppressed catarrh, a third pronounced the ear-drum to be affected, &c.

Applications:—

1. Walking in water daily from two to four minutes, followed by exercise in a warm room or in the open air if the weather be favourable.

2. Every second night a complete lavation, taken from bed.

3. Twice weekly a wet shawl for one hour.

So on for two to three weeks. Should after this

further treatment be necessary, then walking every second day in water, and once a-week a complete lavation.

Epilepsy.

I never allow patients attacked by this illness to relate their case. I only ask them how long they have suffered from it, and whether they have each time been aware of the approach of an attack, by its foreboding symptoms? how old they are? and if their talents and intellectual gifts are still as vigorous as ever, or have already deteriorated?

According to my conviction, this illness too has its seat in the blood, whether it proceed from poverty of blood, diseased unhealthy blood, or disturbed circulation. My opinion is corroborated by the fact that eruptions artificially brought out to the surface, and which, so to say, are the blood's exhalations, have frequently afforded relief to the patient; whereas in cases which prove to be incurable the sufferers are invariably distinguished by a bloated appearance and bluish complexion (agglomerations of unhealthy blood).

If the answers to all my questions were favourable —which is usually the case with young people up to the age of twenty—I then considered their epileptic complaint to be a cramp-like condition, closely allied to St Vitus's dance, and consequently curable. I have been able to bring assistance to many, even such as had inherited the complaint from their parents.

If, however, the patient was unconscious of the approach of his attacks, if already weakness of intellect had begun more or less to set in, then indeed the unfortunate sufferers, who mercifully were seldom aware of the gravity of their condition, had nothing to expect of me.

According to these principles I invariably determined the treatment, which was chiefly directed to the amelioration of the blood. Above all, I endeavoured to induce the patient to brace and harden his system, especially by frequently walking barefoot. In summer I let him take a cold bath occasionally, but never for more than one minute. In winter this bath, slightly warmed, lasted from one to two minutes. Besides this, once weekly a wet shirt dipped in salt water.

The eruptions produced by this last application were treated according to the rules laid down under the head of eruptions. I take care to impress on young people the expediency of dressing in a simple rational manner, and on girls especially the pernicious effect of tight-lacing. The usual diet to be simple and nourishing. The occupations and exercises never forced or strained, but always adapted to the patient's means and strength.

Eruptions.

Under this head we understand all these undefinable skin impurities which sometimes come overnight and are gone next day. We usually attach small importance to these; nevertheless they are often very troublesome, and torment us greatly on chest, back, arms, legs, or other places. This state of things sometimes goes on for years, without the patient being conscious of any serious indisposition, or being hindered in the exercise of his duties. Yet I know many persons whose mind was invariably affected whenever the eruption disappeared, and two cases of raving insanity, in my experience, were the direct consequence of abruptly suppressed eruption. Applications such as those recommended under the headings of Boils and Herpetic Eruptions, caused the rash to reappear on the surface, which had the instantaneous effect of removing the disorder. These eruptions are therefore not so trifling as they appear to be, and may, if neglected, especially as regards cleanliness, have great and serious consequences. Besides mental illness, they may likewise be productive of consumption, liver, kidney, and other complaints. Where any of these has once taken root, it pursues its work of destruction.

I earnestly desire all those who are thus attacked, even should they be yet unconscious of any positive disease, to lose no time in making use of a few light cold-water applications every week. The proper order of taking these would be: cold complete lavations, the Spanish mantle, and the short swathing. Let none be alarmed if, after a time, the eruption comes out stronger than before. That is the best proof of the water's salutary action, and the applications should not be relinquished, but, on the contrary, continued and persevered in.

A farmer related: "For more than two years I have had an eruption on the face and whole body; sometimes there is little to be seen, then again it comes out strongly at particular places. My health is otherwise good, but if this eruption continues to spread, I do not know what may be my fate. I have tried many remedies, but all in vain."

Applications:—

1. Two warm oat-straw baths, twice weekly, with

two changes—that is to say, fifteen minutes in the warm bath, followed each time by one minute in cold water; or in default of a second bath, the body to be vigorously washed over with cold water.

2. Thrice weekly rise from bed and completely wash over the whole body.

3. Daily a pinch of the white bone-powder, as directed in the Pharmacy. Continue thus for three or four weeks, after which go on washing the body once or twice weekly, or else take a semi-bath.

ERYSIPELAS,

or St Anthony's fire, is a formation of poisonous matter between flesh and skin, which seeks to find an outlet. It may appear on the head, foot, arm, or any other part of the body. On whichever spot it arises there is a sense of distension and straining, as though the skin had grown too tight and threatened to burst. It is sometimes long before the eruption appears on the surface, and the patient often suffers great pain. When it breaks out, there first appear isolated fistules filled with a brownish liquid: these increase rapidly, and are so poisonous as to corrode whole parts of the skin. Erysipelas is sometimes dangerous, and may even prove fatal, if the eruption does not succeed in finding an outlet, or when it abruptly disappears from the surface to attack the interior.

I knew a man-servant who got erysipelas on the arm. He made light of it, saying it was but an old woman's complaint. The eruption disappeared, but attacked the brain, and the patient's life was soon at an end.

The principal thing to be observed with regard to erysipelas is, to localise the complaint and keep it from wandering; to expel the unhealthy matter, and avert a conflux of blood towards the affected spot.

Whoever is attacked by erysipelas on the feet, should take a short swathing: this prevents the eruption from spreading upwards. After the short swathing, the leg may be bandaged in wet linen above the affected spot.

Erysipelas may, however, be attacked directly; this is done by dipping soft linen in warm water and applying it to the place, secured and covered by a dry cloth. This serves to dissolve and expel the poison.

For erysipelas on the arm, a short swathing should first be taken to divert the blood from above. Then follows a shawl, to be renewed as often as required according to the heat. The eruption may here also be treated directly as above.

Erysipelas on the head will best be averted by an upper compress, in combination with a throat swathing. When these two applications have been employed once or twice, then the affected spot may be treated first with warm, and afterwards with cold water.

"My husband has got erysipelas: the whole face is swollen and fiery red; he has violent fever; the red colour spreads over the whole face; little fistules are to be seen everywhere, and his moanings are dreadful to hear,"—so lamented a wife to me. "Take quickly a shawl dipped in warm water," I ordered; "let him keep it on three-quarters of an hour, then renew it by dipping in fresh water. This process to be repeated three times. Three to four hours later place a cold compress on the lower body for three hours but renew at the end of every hour. Three hours later, when the compress has been removed, let the patient lie for an hour upon a wet sheet folded together three or four fold. These three applications can be repeated in the same sequence until the heat is entirely withdrawn, and the unhealthy matter removed. Nothing is to be applied to the inflamed spots, except to wash them gently from time to time with lukewarm water whenever the tension of the skin is unbearable. If the thirst be great, water or sugar-water is the best beverage—always, however, imbibed in small portions."

Another way to cure erysipelas is to give the patient a shawl twice daily, each time for three hours (renew after one hour), and in the intervals to wash over the body with vinegar-and-water every three-quarters of an hour as long as the fever continues to be strong. When the fever decreases, every two to three hours will be sufficient, and later only once or twice a-day. The water, which at first may be lukewarm, should afterwards be exchanged for cold.

In both these ways I have cured many cases of erysipelas.

Eyes, Cataract of the.

An official brought me a boy nine years of age, whose eyes were affected. Both eyes were so bad that only with difficulty could the boy walk alone. "How come you to me?" I asked. "My child," replied the father, "was for a long time in a sanatory establishment for eye-complaints, but was dismissed with the declaration that his was an incurable case of cataract. That is dreadful, to be blind at the age of nine!"

One eye was already so much dimmed that the pupil could scarcely be discerned, and for the child it was utter darkness. On the other eye there lay a cloud; and as the outer disc of the sun, when about to set behind a bank of clouds, shines out once more, so too here a narrow strip of the once healthy eye shone out a last time before extinction.

The unfortunate boy suffered not only from the eyes, as I saw at the first glance: his whole little system was weakened and impaired, decayed through and through apparently; no life, no appetite, emaciated, and with dry scurfy skin. The body, then, not only the eyes, is diseased; let us first seek to cure this, perhaps then the eyes will open by-and-by.

We began by removing the spectacles he had hitherto worn. The boy was made to walk as much as possible barefoot in the wet grass or on wet stones; and his back, chest, and abdomen were vigorously washed over once or twice a-day. After some time the lavations were exchanged for semi-baths, and these again in turn for whole baths, which never lasted above one minute. Between these were alternately employed swathings, or the wet shirt dipped in a solution of salt and water, and applied for one and a half hour. All these applications had the object of bracing the system and inciting it to renewed life and action.

For acting directly on the eyes themselves, I employed several kinds of eye-water. First, aloe water (a pinch of aloe powder boiled for a few minutes in half a pint of water), with which the eyes were thoroughly washed out, especially inside the lids, from three to five times daily. Aloe dissolves, cleanses, and heals.

This aloe water was followed up later by water of alum (two pinches of alum dissolved in half a pint of water), and applied like the former, three or four times daily. Alum is corrosive and cleansing in its effects. Finally, I made use of honey eye-water (half a spoonful of honey boiled for five minutes in half a pint of water), and employed from three to five times daily, especially upon the inner eye. The boy throve so markedly under this treatment, that from week to week his strength increased, his appearance became fresher, healthier, and more blooming; mind and body alike gradually returned to their normal condition. The long-closed eyes reopened and sparkled anew, to the inexpressible joy of the happy parents. The boy now sees as well as any of his schoolfellows. No one would deem that he had ever been in such a wretched plight.

I am firmly persuaded that the woful state of the eyes were but a reflection and a consequence of the yet more woful body; and as from a decayed trunk the leaves and blossoms must necessarily wither and fall, so in a diseased body, the eyes could not be otherwise than affected also. When the sap of life is renewed within the trunk, then twigs and branches begin to sprout afresh and put forth new leaves and blossoms.

EYES, CATARRH OF.

A well-known military doctor said to me thirty years ago: "Catarrh is an evil out of which almost any other disease may arise—as nervous fever, typhus, dysentery, consumption, &c. Let every one therefore brace his constitution, so as to render it impervious to the manifold chances of catching cold. Whoever has a catarrh should not rest until it be shaken off."

Blindness and misery are synonymous, and every ocular disease must therefore be regarded as a source of misery. Our eyes are the most precious jewels we possess—but of them we have only two—and even to lose one is an irreparable loss. Let every one therefore be careful. Eye complaints are to be found in persons of all age, sex, and station.

In the majority of cases, the disease proceeds directly from the body. In healthy persons the superfluous secretions are removed by perspiration, breathing, and other means; but in the unhealthy these secretions accumulate in the body, head, &c. Whatever accumulates in the head is apt to seek an outlet through the eyes, which, being infinitely delicate and tender, are easily injured by the sharp corrosive moisture. This is the cause of the eye-burning from which so many people suffer. Cure is only to be effected by the removal of the pernicious moisture. The eye itself is healthy, and only suffers from its propinquity to the unwholesome matter.

Many eyes are affected to the degree of partial blindness; with others it resembles a slight veil or mist; others, again, seem to see sparks or dancing specks. All these various effects proceed from the same course. Remove the poisonous matter, strengthen the weakened eye, and it is cured. An example may serve to elucidate my meaning.

Antonia, a little girl five years old, looks very pale. Her face is bloated, and whole appearance sickly. The child has inflamed eyes, and cannot bear the light. Appetite and sleep are impaired, and the child cries very much. What is to be done?

Wrap the child's body up to the armpits daily in a

towel dipped in lukewarm water wherein oat-straw has been boiled. Over this wet towel wrap a second dry one. If this is done before the child's usual sleeping-time, it will probably soon go to sleep, in which case it should not be disturbed. If, however, it does not sleep, the wet wrapper must be kept on for an hour. This proceeding to be continued for a week. In the second week prepare a warm bath with decoction of oat-straw (86° to 91° F.), and let it remain therein from fifteen to twenty minutes. In the last minute pour rapidly over the child the contents of a small watering-can, of plain not too cold water, and then dress quickly. This cold affusion after each warm bath is very important. The warm bath fulfils the object of dissolving and removing the unhealthy matter; while the cold affusion serves to strengthen and close the pores. Every second or third day the bath should be repeated. The child will soon feel fresher, stronger, and healthier, and the eyes will be clearer.

Should the anxious mother desire a direct remedy for the eye, let her take a piece of alum, as large as four grains of barley, dissolve this in half a pint of water, and wash the child's eyes with it three or four times daily. Soon everything will be well. Even when the complaint has been removed, let the mother continue for some time to give the child once weekly a bath, or a wrapping on alternate weeks.

William, a boy of nine years, had an eye complaint. He could no longer read, hardly even distinguish people's faces, and was more than half blind. More than 400 marks had already been spent on his eyes, but neither doctor nor apothecary was able to help him. Not only the eyes but likewise the whole system was gravely impaired; hands and feet were always cold, the stomach without appetite, the body emaciated, the whole figure mournful and depressed.

In four months William was completely cured, both eyes and body. Twice a-week he took a warm bath. Four times weekly a shirt dipped in salt water from an hour to an hour and a half. In addition to this, I made the boy walk frequently barefoot in wet grass or in the rain. After the lapse of the first four weeks, William continued to bathe three to four times weekly for one minute only, and with the temperature reduced (66° F.), each bath succeeded by exercise. Twice daily he washed the eyes in water mixed with alum. This second course of treatment lasted several weeks. By degrees, as the general tone of the system was restored, so too in equal measure the eyesight improved. The eyes soon looked out of the boy's fresh and healthy face, as clear and sparkling as though they had never been affected.

Christina, twenty-four years old, though fresh and blooming, is yet scarcely ever free from eye complaint. She has too much blood in the head, too little in the feet, for which reason she always suffers from cold feet.

Christina takes every day a lukewarm foot-bath, mixed with salt and ashes. This draws down the blood from the head. Three times a-week she takes a semi-bath reaching to the armpits, half a minute. At work she mostly goes barefoot. The pressure of blood to the head gradually decreased and stopped altogether, and the eye complaint disappeared.

Fever.

Anthony comes into the room and relates: "With difficulty I have contrived to mount the stairs. My strength is quite broken, and twice I have fallen down. I have also a dreadful headache, and am alternately icy cold and burning hot. Sometimes I feel a stabbing pain, as if lightning were darting about inside my body."

Application: "Go home, Anthony, lie down at once in bed, and when you are quite warm wash over the whole body with cold water, and without drying return to bed. Repeat this washing every two hours, and when you begin to perspire strongly, and the perspiration has lasted half an hour, then wash again."

Anthony returned on the third day, and related: "I feel much better; I have sweated profusely several times.. Cold and heat have disappeared, and the headache has ceased. The appetite begins to return. I feel well, but weary."

Anthony continued to wash about ten times within fourteen days, and was then able to rejoice in perfect health. He is about forty years old.

Gout.

In manuring a field it is bad to heap the dung too thickly on any particular spot, for instead of promoting fruitfulness this merely gives rise to fetid swamps wherein nothing can thrive. In the same way excessive and superfluous nourishment of the body produces gout, which is mostly to be traced to overindulgence in eating and drinking. Other causes of gout may be great exertion, wettings, catching cold,

&c. Acute gout torments many persons; chronic gout innumerable ones. Some it attacks in the toes, others in the head; some externally, many internally.

Persons of simple habits, and who are not over-weakened by the complaint, I can easily and readily cure; but I seldom have any such illusion with regard to the more distinguished class of gout patients. They are a heavy burden, and mostly incurable by water, for they will not obey orders, and suffer alike from effeminacy and dread of cold water; were it not so, they would be as easily cured as the others.

A gentleman of position suffered four weeks from violent foot pains. He was cured the first time by sweating; but a year later the complaint returned, and chained him to bed for twelve weeks. It burned much and he sweated much, but this time the moisture failed to bring relief. He sent to consult me, saying he would do anything in order to be freed from this dreadful illness. In a few weeks the chief cure was accomplished. As water poured upon quicklime inflates and breaks it up, so here, too, the gout tumours disappeared under the various applications. Later the patient continued to employ cold water from time to time, in one or the other form, and as far as I am aware, the former complaint never troubled him again. The reader can learn the applications from the following case:—

A priest sent a message to say that his feet were burning like living fire—he was almost in despair. What should he do? I advised him to infuse hay-flowers in hot water for some minutes, then, pressing out the moisture, to place the flowers on a linen cloth and wrap then well round both feet. After two hours he was to dip again the hay-flowers in the decoction, and replace as before. It is a matter of indifference whether the hay-flowers be applied cold or lukewarm the second time. The sick priest did this for several days. After the first day the principal pains had ceased; in two or three days he was completely free of suffering.

In default of hay-flowers oat-straw may be used.

I must warn here against a common error. As soon as the feet have ceased to hurt, the patient often imagines himself to be completely cured. It were a great mistake to terminate here the cure, which must be followed up by at least some water applications, in order to expel the unhealthy matter from the body. It is best to employ the Spanish mantle two or three times weekly during the first three weeks (for one and a half to two hours). In the following month some warm baths with hay-flowers or oat-straw decoction, and with threefold transition into cold water.

A day labourer had acquired a serious gout complaint. Three times weekly he went into a sack dipped in a hot oat-straw infusion. Twice in the week he took a hot pine-tree bath (106° to 111° F.), each time with threefold transition into the cold water. Every second night a complete cold lavation taken from bed. After three weeks he was nearly cured, but continued to employ the oat-straw sack once or twice on alternate weeks with the aforementioned warm bath. Soon with renewed strength he resumed his labours, which he is still to-day able to perform.

Gravel and Stone Complaint.

Gravel and stone are often formed in the bladder or kidneys. Those who have beheld sufferers from gravel, or have themselves been attacked with this complaint, know how dreadful are these pains. Cure by water is infallible and painless, therefore always the simplest and best.

Oat-straw baths here occupy the first place. Oat-straw (or in default of this shave-grass or sour hay) is boiled for half an hour, and the decoction poured into a warm bath (100° F.) In this bath let the patient stay one hour, concluding it by a vigorous cold lavation. Three such baths in the week may be taken. Alongside of these, two or three short swathings or else compresses, of four to six fold linen, on the affected parts, will do excellent service. Both applications are of course to be taken in bed. These serve to loosen and dissolve the gravel-stones in bladder and kidneys, and expel them. Teas also play an important part in this malady. First and foremost stands tea of oats. Oats are boiled for half an hour, and of the infusion two cupfuls daily are drunk. Of more potent effect is tea of oat-straw, prepared like the former. Shave-grass tea is hardly to be surpassed. I will still mention rose-hips, of which, likewise, when boiled, a very efficacious tea may be made, which, however, must be drunk for some length of time. Experience has taught me that this rose-hip tea prevents the further formation of stone or gravel. The aforementioned applications should be pursued for two or three weeks as directed, and for the subsequent three or four weeks reduced by one-half. The blessing of the greatest of all physicians will soon dispel the illness.

A gentleman who acted under my directions told

me that within a few weeks he had expelled several thousand particles of stone.

Another gentleman suffered so dreadfully from stone and gravel that the corrosive juices had penetrated to the feet, and produced there innumerable little boils. A sensation of itching and burning often pervaded the whole body. Thirty baths within a year, the Spanish mantle used two or three times weekly, and the aforementioned teas, completely removed the complaint and its irksome effects.[1]

Headache.

A gentleman of distinction was afflicted with a peculiar sort of headache. It used regularly to begin at 7 A.M., and continue till sunset, and was so painful that he could neither read nor write while it lasted. At night there was no trace of pain, the headache had completely disappeared, provided he had not over-fatigued himself by mental work. The painful spot was on the left side of the forehead, and about the size of half-a-crown. The pain not only affected the head, but extended to the whole body, so that he visibly declined in appearance as in strength. The most celebrated doctors were consulted, and one cold-water establishment was visited, without apparent effect.

[1] Quite recently knot-grass (*Polygonum aviculare*) has been employed by Pfarrer Kneipp for this complaint. A cupful of knot-grass tea, taken morning and evening, in combination with a daily sitz-bath of shave-grass decoction, will have the best results. For further use, the sitz-bath should be continued from twice to thrice weekly, or else every second day a back and lower affusion may be applied.—Translator's note.

A visit to Meran brought him temporary relief, and he deemed himself cured; but hardly had the patient returned to town when, on the following morning, at exactly 7 o'clock, the old headache punctually reappeared, to his inexpressible disappointment and vexation. At last the gentleman, urged by some friends, resolved to consult me. His appearance was sickly and much emaciated. After describing his complaint, he added that he was seldom free from catarrh, and possessed but small latent heat.

All these symptoms led me to conclude that not one particular spot in the head alone was here affected, but rather the whole system. In accordance with this presumption, I therefore directed the applications towards the whole body independent of the head, which received no special attention. The simplest means of hardening, combined with a few lavations, sufficed to effect the cure and restore circulation, perspiration, and digestion to their normal regularity. It was the same old story which, however, cannot be sufficiently often repeated.

The result proved the correctness of my opinion regarding the headache. In about six weeks the whole system rejoiced in unimpaired health, and the dreaded headache no longer put in an appearance at 7 o'clock.

A man related:—

"I am thirty-five years old, have continual headache, and sometimes feel so weak that I can scarcely bear it. I have pains in back and chest,—most painful of all in the nape of the neck, where I feel a permanent cramp-like contraction. My hair is falling out profusely, and if this continues half a year I shall be completely bald. Hands and feet are mostly cold, and I have no appetite."

Applications:—

1. A wet shirt dipped in salt water.
2. Thrice in the week a complete lavation taken from bed.
3. A wet shirt thrice in the week.
4. Daily a pinch of white bone-powder.

After two months the man returned to me and declared himself to be completely cured: he only suffered occasionally from very slight and transitory pains, where the former violent sufferings had been. His bodily weight had increased by 10 lb.

Headache, Nervous.

A man aged forty-five came lamenting to me and began: "The doctor pronounces my complaint to be a nervous headache. I can never be without a head bandage; I feel an intolerable pressure on the back of the head, now to the right, now to the left. When the pain comes to the back, then I get violent palpitation of the heart for several hours. My appetite is sometimes quite gone; I suffer so much from giddiness that I cannot walk alone, for which reason my wife was obliged to come here with me. But worse than all my pains are my mental sufferings. I feel so depressed that I often long for death to come."

This gentleman was tolerably stout, the complexion sallow, the body much inflated.

In thirteen days order was restored to the system. The bodily weight had decreased, headache and giddiness disappeared; sleep and appetite had returned along with good spirits. The applications were as follows:—

1. On the first day an upper affusion and knee affusion in the forenoon; back affusion and walking in water afternoon.

2. On the second day, in the forenoon back affusion; later, water-walking. Afternoon, again back affusion, and later, knee affusion.

3. On the third day, upper affusion and knee affusion in the forenoon. Complete affusion, and later a semi-bath, in the afternoon.

The patient being strong and stout, was able to endure four applications daily.

Heart Complaints.

In the restless excitable times in which we live, innumerable persons are supposed to be attacked by nerve, stomach, or heart complaints. These are the three scapegoats upon which all misdeeds are foisted. These conclusions are mostly erroneous, as experience has taught me, and amongst a hundred cases in which the patients believed their heart to be attacked, of very few only this proved to be the case. The heart, though one of the strongest and healthiest organs, may sometimes be momentarily affected by passing influences, just as the healthiest cat will cry out if we pinch its tail. The best clock will stop going if we remove the weights; it were then folly to say the clock is bad. The most wonderful flute gives out no tune if I stop up the holes or allow it to rust. The healthiest heart can likewise be obstructed in its action if there be present in the body a foe which, so to say, throttles it. Seek out this foe, and remove certain pernicious influences, and there will remain no trace of the heart complaint.

A gentleman of position had suffered for many years, and could only pursue his vocation with great difficulty. An unusual sense of anxiety aggravated his sufferings. The smallest event caused him palpitation, excitement, and fear. Those around him had to be very careful of their words, for unexpected joy or sorrow always brought about disordered action of the heart. The rooms had to be heated summer and winter, and the temperature exactly regulated to a particular degree. The most celebrated doctors had been consulted, and were unanimous in declaring the patient, in addition to affected lungs and liver, and piles, to be afflicted with an organic heart complaint which might at any moment terminate in heart-stroke. Eventually this gentleman died and was dissected. What was the result? That lungs, liver, and heart were perfectly sound, but that agglomerations of fat had formed upon heart and chest. He therefore died from want of blood. The blood came to fail, having been absorbed by the formation of muscles and fat. This was related to me by a doctor who was present at the dissection, and who remarked, "Here we have another instance of science being completely deceived."

A young lady came to me and begged for help. She related thus: "I have successfully gone through a course as musical teacher, and have taught music in a convent for six years. Now I suffer so much from headache that I can scarcely stand the sound of an instrument—either organ, violin, or pianoforte. Even the altar hand-bell causes a stabbing pain in the head.

The doctors call my condition a nerve and heart complaint. If I had been healthy, I should have been accepted in the convent; but now I am without vocation and almost without bread, and suffer indescribable mental and bodily pain."

I answered: "I cannot help you. You must seek for assistance elsewhere."

To her question as to why I gave such a hard answer just to her, I replied frankly: "You, as a town young lady, with such musical and linguistic accomplishments, would never obey my orders; otherwise, your unhappy condition is curable." She answered resolutely, "I shall do what you ask, in order to recover my health." And she kept her word. For ten days I sent her out with a maid-servant—it was in the month of March—into the meadows, where she walked barefoot. Daily, in order to accustom her gradually to the cold, a warm foot-bath and an upper affusion. Instead of the warm foot-bath, after six days, she daily knelt in water reaching to the pit of the stomach. Also field labour was prescribed, so far as strength and practice allowed. After eighteen days, the young lady returned to a benefactor who had assisted her musical studies, and had also advised the cold-water cure. There she continued the applications, as well as the now congenial field labours. Piano and violin were exchanged for the spade, rake, and hoe. The more the body gained in vigour, in the same measure the heart and nervous symptoms disappeared. In four months she was completely cured, and the freshness and health of her childhood were hers again.

A theological student came and asked me what he

should do. His whole system seemed decayed, and the doctors had declared that, amongst other things, he had a heart complaint. He had wished to become a priest, but with these headaches and palpitations this was out of the question. Everything which he heard and saw seemed to him like a dream.

I advised the patient rationally to brace his body. This would do him no harm, for he was well built. Later on he could adopt the profession for which he felt most inclination.

After a few weeks he was able to resume his studies, received holy orders in two years, and few of his comrades were his match in strength and health.

Every morning the young gentleman walked for half an hour in the wet dewy grass, and daily stood in the water up to the pit of the stomach, with a lavation of the upper body. In rainy weather, light works were substituted for his favourite walks in the forest. Later on, by way of strengthening, he received frequent upper affusions daily, one or two, in alternation with semi-baths. Head and heart complaint soon vanished with the gradual increase of his general strength.

Herpetic Eruptions.

Many thousands of men are tormented by herpetic eruptions, whether they choose to acknowledge it or not. These troublesome parasites and vampires are fond of lodging themselves under the hair, on the back, chest, &c. Sometimes they do not shun the light of day, and fasten themselves like leeches on the arms, feet, and especially between the toes and fingers. These eruptions may either be hereditary, or else the consequence of bad food and beverages, which ruin the secretions; not infrequently, too, they are caused by a disordered mode of life.

It is dangerous to attack this unclean visitor with violent weapons (either external or internal), such as quicksilver, arsenic, &c. The eruption may indeed thus readily be subdued, but the consequences of violently suppressing it are often worse than the actual complaint, apart from the injury which sharp corrosive applications occasion to the skin.

My rules for healing this disease are as follows:—

Outwardly I only permit lukewarm water to be used, in order to wash away the dirt. Everything else can only do harm.

Food and drink for these patients should be light and easily digestible; simple, yet sufficiently nourishing to arrest the process of forming new unhealthy secretions, and improving the existing ones. Everything acid or salt should be avoided. The water applications are as follows: On the first day let the patient take a head vapour-bath and a lower swathing; on the second day a vapour foot-bath and a lower swathing; on the third morning, again, a Spanish mantle, and a short swathing in the afternoon. The fourth day should be a day of rest, all applications being suspended. On the fifth day let the patient remain in bed, and rapidly wash over the body with cold water every two hours. Should he be prevented from staying in bed, this may be replaced by three lavations in the day, followed up by exercise. The applications are to be modified and gradually lessened in proportion as the herpetic eruption begins to cease, and the formation of the new skin progresses.

Let another remark find place here: herpetic eruptions are sometimes classified as wet or dry eruptions. For either kind the same course of treatment is to be observed. The two complaints are really identical, —the dry eruption, in which the moisture is trifling, and soon assumes the appearance of incrustations, being the lighter form of the disease; whereas wet eruptions, which are apt to pass into running sores, are graver, more troublesome, and dangerous in their effects.

The consequences of violently suppressed herpetic eruptions are incalculable. The serious diseases to which they often directly give rise may lead to a slow decline, often ending in death, or, still worse, in insanity.

A theological student had on his left cheek a round disc, as though drawn with a mathematical instrument. It was covered with a crust which, like a lid, lay over the raw flesh, and was raised from time to time in order to let out two or three drops of matter. This gentleman's face was full; on the head some little fistules were to be seen. The patient had consulted several doctors and tried various remedies, but without success.

My question as to whether he had received a wound was answered in the negative: this thing had come spontaneously, without apparent cause. I was now clear as to his condition. The poisonous matter proceeded from the body.

Fifteen to twenty years ago, many persons used to make for themselves what they called *Fontanellen* (little fountains) by opening out a small hole in the flesh of arm or leg. This hole, which was never allowed to close, served as issue for all the unhealthy matter contained in the body, and was in a continual state of suppuration. In the above-mentioned case vigorous Nature had herself constructed the aperture, supplying it with a suitable covering.

For seventeen days the patient had to take a head vapour-bath every second day; likewise as often a vapour foot-bath. These were assisted by the Spanish mantle and the short swathing, in such manner that each day two or three applications took place. Tea of sage, wormwood, and mint assisted the process internally. Beneath the crust a delicate skin began soon to form, the surest sign that the dissolving and expelling process was accomplished. After three weeks it was no longer possible to discern which cheek had been the affected one.

Hoarseness.

A girl aged eleven had so completely lost her voice for several months that she could only make herself understood with great difficulty in a hoarse croaking fashion. Her complexion was pale, the eyes bluish, and her appearance emaciated and nerveless. The latent heat had disappeared, as also the appetite, except for a little beer or wine.

Within two months the girl was completely cured by means of the following applications:—

1. Walking barefoot in wet grass from two to four times daily.
2. Three to four times weekly a wet shawl.
3. Four sitz-baths every week.
4. In warm weather, during the last three weeks, bathing in sunny water three times weekly.

The diet consisted of plain homely fare, especially milk, taken in table-spoonfuls, one every hour.

I received news that the girl is now quite well and healthy.

A priest suffered from hoarseness, which regularly set in from October to May. He tried everything, consulted various doctors, but in vain. The complaint remained fixed during fourteen years. At last he sought help from me, and got it in a wonderfully short time.

The gentleman was made to stand every day in water reaching above the knees, and simultaneously to hold his arms in water. Besides this he undertook complete lavations, mostly on rising in the morning, or at night from bed.

After twelve days this ancient complaint had vanished completely, and has not reappeared during sixteen years.

A proof of how thoroughly water can cure.

HYPOCHONDRIASIS.

I have always the sincerest compassion for hypochondriacs, whose condition is often ridiculed and made light of by thoughtless persons. Really these sufferers deserve our greatest pity and sympathy. On beholding one of these I always ask myself the question, "Was this hypochondriac once a normal individual? Was there a time when he thought sensibly and worked diligently?" If the answer be affirmative, then it were folly on my part to believe that nothing is the matter with this man, that he merely assumes these follies in order to torment himself and others. Rather, I tell myself, some transformation must have taken place in mind or body; something must be seriously amiss in order to cause these symptoms. And then I say to myself, "Let us seek to heal that which has changed, to restore the former healthy condition, and the hypochondriasis will cease of its own accord." Often the best and most active persons, who have fatigued their minds by over-study, fall into this mental condition.

The seat of hypochondriasis, as of every other kind of mental disease, should in my opinion be sought in the sick body. Seek to rouse the indolent system, to fortify whatever is weak, restore the blood to its normal circulation, and the cure will be complete.

I knew a man gifted with brilliant talents. Many years he lived happily in his vocation, doing with ease and enthusiasm as much work as two others. Suddenly he turned hypochondriac, to the extent of totally neglecting his profession, shunning and fearing everything, and flying from all society.

Instead of help and sympathy, of which he stood more in need than others, daily and hourly he was met with ridicule, and the contemptuous judgment, "You are just a hypochondriac! There is no help for you!" Was this not sufficient to crush any man?

Strange to say, this gentleman had already visited two different hydropathic establishments, whose treatment had only increased the complaint. The applications were too rough, too violent. Instead of helping to build up the crumbling edifice, they accelerated its ruin.

In this case I had the opportunity of convincing myself that water, when employed in the mildest form, really achieves the greatest results. That such a complaint cannot, however, be removed in a few days, is self-evident.

The most suitable water applications consist in complete and partial lavations, in baths (especially sitz-baths), short swathings, and finally in whole baths.

Inflammation, General Remarks.

A boy scarcely yet able to walk sees how the mother has struck a light. He does not rest until he too has found a match to make fire with. He succeeds in so doing, and the little criminal soon contrives to burn down the house, with everything it contains.

How many men lie now in the churchyard whose illness began by a tiny spark of diseased matter, which spread conflagration throughout the body as the spark turned to a flame! The blood, converging from all sides to the affected spot, acted like oil upon the flames. Proper means of extinguishing were not resorted to, and the soul's luckless habitation was suffered to perish miserably. Thousands of animals are thus annually destroyed. Thousands of men meet with a similar fate. How quickly this sometimes happens! Your throat has caught fire at one tiny spot—it is inflamed. A rough breeze chances to come, and fans the spark to a flame; the veins supply more combustible matter, and in a few hours the whole throat is on fire. Is it not so? What should we do? What do the people do when there is a fire? They give the alarm, and seek to save what may yet be saved. Then, if there still be time, they seek to remove all combustible matter from the neighbourhood of the flames, and set to spouting water with the fire-engine. These hints we should understand and take to heart.

Whenever an inflammation has appeared, we should seek to arrest the conflux of blood to the affected part. We thus can save the yet healthy blood from becoming inflamed. Simultaneously we must act upon the seat of the evil, in order to dispel the agglomeration of blood.

To return to the subject of throat inflammation. Touch the feet and see if they be not icy cold. This is often the case. The blood has left the feet to fly to the seat of inflammation in the throat. Wrap the feet in linen cloths dipped in vinegar-and-water. Returning warmth will soon be felt. The foot-swathing draws down the blood, and already some of the combustible matter has been removed. Then seek to lead back the blood to its proper seat in the abdomen. This is done by placing similar cloths, dipped in vinegar-and-water, on the lower body. These compresses should be renewed whenever the cloths have absorbed much heat. By this time a good deal of inflammable matter will have been expelled, and the throat itself may be next attacked. Dip a cloth in the very coldest water, and wind round the neck, but do not let the cloth become too hot, which would only tend to produce fresh heat in the body, and so defeat its own end.

My thirty years' experience has taught me to reject the practice of Priessnitz and his followers, of keeping on the compress the whole night undisturbed, having frequently found its effect to be more pernicious than salutary. The compress should, cn the contrary, be changed as often as it has absorbed heat. The patient's own feeling will usually be the best counsellor as to how often this should be done.

INFLUENZA.[1]

Though much has been written about influenza, no remedy has yet been suggested by means of which this malady may be quickly and surely cured. The germs of this illness are believed to be in the atmosphere, and then it is with influenza as with other epidemics which are conveyed by the air. In my opinion, influenza is almost identical with the complaint universally known as "Grippe" among the people. It is mostly caused by a rapid change of temperature from cold to warm, or *vice versâ,* and living as we do, in a degenerate age, many persons are apt to be affected by these abrupt transitions of nature. The cold of the atmosphere comes in collision with the body's latent heat, and in the ensuing struggle the latter is often vanquished, more especially by reason of the heavy artificial coverings worn about head and throat. The throat is attacked by inflammation, which spreads to head and chest, finally to the entire body. I will here illustrate the symptoms of this illness by means of an example.

A man-servant came to me and said: "Yesterday evening I was quite well, and felt not the slightest symptoms of indisposition. To-day I am half paralysed, so that I am scarcely able to walk: my legs tremble under me; I have a dreadful headache, and am quite dizzy. In the throat there is such a burning and stabbing that I cannot swallow."

To the man thus suddenly attacked by influenza I gave the following advice:—

[1] At the time when the influenza epidemic broke out in the winter of 1889-90, Pfarrer Kneipp published these directions for subduing the malady.—Translator's note.

"Go to bed at once; wash your neck, chest, and whole upper body with very cold water, and tie a dry linen towel about your neck. Cover yourself up warmly, but not over heavily. Continue to wash yourself in this manner every hour for ten hours. Then completely wash over the entire body with cold water as rapidly as possible." After this complete lavation, there broke out such a violent perspiration that the patient was drenched with it all over as he lay in bed, and with this perspiration the last remains of the disease were likewise swept away: the patient had regained his former peasant vigour.

Some persons may be inclined to ask how these simple remedies sufficed to cure the disease. Listen, readers: The cold had conquered in the throat, and occasioned inflammation. Hardly had this formed, than the blood all rushed to the seat of conflagration. There was an undue conflux of blood to head and throat; the extremities were cold and bloodless. By means of the lavations the pores of the skin were opened, and new heat restored, especially through the swathing of the dry towel. This caused an effluence from head and throat, by which means all unwholesome matter was drawn from the system. Internally a spoonful of water was administered every hour to the patient. This likewise served to dissolve and expel. As washing and swathing with the linen cloth on the upper body, in like manner the complete lavation acted upon the whole body, opening the pores and increasing the latent heat. The warm bed thus removed all unwholesome matter contained in the system, and eighteen hours sufficed completely to expel this unwelcome guest.

INSANITY.

How fearful, is it not, when some one is afflicted by darkness of the mind! when man is no longer man, but rather resembles the unreasoning beast! Fifty, forty, thirty years ago, mental diseases were the exception; to-day (it is a well-known fact) their number is terribly on the increase. The mad-houses —however numerous they may be—are crowded, and in some places whole new suburbs have been built outside the towns for receiving the insane. There are, however, many persons afflicted with partial insanity, who suffer much, and whose condition receives little attention and help. In truth I may say that I have been able to assist a large number of these unfortunates, who came to seek relief and solace of me, and with peculiar love and care I have always felt myself especially drawn to these neglected and hopeless beings. They were not ill enough for the asylum, but unfit for any responsible employment. Indescribable, unspeakable, innumerable, and various are the troubles of these disordered minds. As on a summer day, in the burning heat at noon, the midges swarm most wildly in the air, so the most incongruous thoughts keep thronging and revolving in the heated brain of these poor creatures. Some of them have taken a sudden aversion to their formerly beloved occupation; others refuse to pray. Fear or hatred of men has taken possession of the one, hatred of his own self pursues the other; hankering after suicide afflicts many, &c. The heads and their contents are as different as are the poor individuals from each other.

In every patient who came to consult me, in the

course of my thirty years' practice, I was able to discover some reason for his complaint. Either the disease was hereditary, or else it was caused by some direct bodily complaint; often, too, from a disordered mode of life.

Upon one point I must lay stress, as deceptions are apt to occur. Those who treat such complaints should strive to remain as cool-headed and impartial as possible in judging a case. I cannot sufficiently warn against the foolish rashness with which many are apt to jump to the conclusion that some supernatural, more especially diabolical, influence must be here implicated. Even in cases when any one might have believed Satan himself to be in possession of the patient's body, a simple cold gush was often sufficient to chase away the devil.

In my whole practice I never met with a single case in which natural means, properly employed, were not effective. I hold firmly to my faith, and to the doctrine of the supernatural, as to my lifeboat, and, so God help me, I will never give up a hair's-breadth of my convictions. But never would I give a handle to the enemies of my faith, by exposing my religion to derisive attacks.

Those whom this may concern, will understand what I mean. Here is an example:—

A brother brought to me his sister, who declared that in her breast resided the evil spirit. She knew much about the devil, but he knew all about her, even her most inmost thoughts; he governed, led, and commanded her: her brother was a fool, stupider still was the priest, and the doctor the greatest fool of the three. Why? "Because they always say I should get a new head, give up my follies, and obey them. But if once the devil has got possession of me," continued the patient, "then the head is no longer able to govern." I can scarcely describe how violently and wildly the unfortunate girl stormed and railed against the three persons she had named.

If they had had the sense, knowing her condition, to be silent, they would not thus have excited her, and I should have had an easier part to play.

With such patients everything depends upon the manner of treatment. I therefore refrained from contradicting the girl, and merely said, "Yes, verily, your interior is in a sad condition." This satisfied the patient, and I had won her to my side by inspiring confidence, as her answer showed: "If one refuses to believe that the devil is inside me, then naturally he is incapable of driving him out."

This confidence once gained, half the battle is won, and the patient more than half cured. She took submissively the medicines I gave, and applied the water as I directed. In six weeks she was completely cured. It may interest some readers to know what had really been the matter with this person. Her appearance was very wild. Her features were sunken, the hands cold, the feet still colder; she felt a heavy pressure on the chest, and aversion to all food. All blood seemed to have concentrated itself on the chest. The first task consisted in regulating the circulation, and restoring equal warmth and general activity to the system. In order to attain this, the patient was made to stand daily twice in water reaching above the calves, for two minutes each time, after which she took strong exercise until the feet were thoroughly warm; likewise twice daily she held her whole arms in water for two minutes, succeeded by exercise as before. Twice daily, when lying in bed, chest, back, and lower body were vigorously washed over with vinegar-and-water. These applications were continued for fourteen days. The violent excitement subsided, although the devil still continued to haunt her disordered head. The sunken features began to revive. After fourteen days I increased the strength of the applications. The patient received lower swathings, alternately with semi-baths (only half a minute) and the Spanish mantle. These three applications were continued for about three weeks. After the third week the cure consisted in one complete lavation, and one short swathing of one hour weekly. In this manner the *quondam* devil was expelled, and the former excitement exchanged for undisturbed peace and calm.

Poor parents brought to me their boy, aged ten, and related as follows: "As often as the church bells begin to ring, the boy breaks out into the wildest ravings and curses that we have ever heard. He continues to curse and swear till he sees the last church-goer enter the church, then he stops. As soon, however, as service is ended, and the congregation begins to flock out, he begins again to curse, and curses on until there is no one more to be seen. When we pray, then he curses, and when we stop praying then he also stops. It is fearful, your reverence! Whatever we try is of no use, and all admonitions only serve to increase his violence. He once seized his mother in both arms as with claws, and shook her so violently that we never thought a boy could possess so much strength. Many doctors have been consulted, but they availed nothing. He was also blessed (by a priest), but that only made him curse the more violently," &c.

The boy had a singular appearance—an unhealthy complexion, his features wildly distorted, his hair stood on end like a hedgehog's quills. When I endeavoured to feel his hand, he wanted to spring at my face. Two priests who had seen this terrible condition said, "Whoever believes in possession of the devil must say, This is it."

I judged the complaint to be a purely natural one—nor was I mistaken. In six weeks' time the poor child was completely cured. I made the boy put on daily for one to one and a half hour a shirt dipped in salt and water, and likewise daily caused him to be washed over with a mixture of vinegar-and-water. This was continued for fourteen days. In the third week the applications were as follows: On the first day the wet salt shirt as above directed; on the second a warm bath (95° F.) for half an hour, terminated by a plunge in cold water of half a minute; on the third day a complete lavation. So on for two weeks further. In the fifth week one wet shirt was sufficient, and in the sixth and last, a warm bath, succeeded by a rapid cold plunge.

The cure was quickly accomplished, the cold body became warm again, the lost appetite returned, and all uncanny symptoms disappeared.

Some readers may ask, "Why does not the pastor employ cold douches for these complaints, such as are in general use for violent maniacs in many madhouses?" My humble opinion is, that in order to capture a fox the hunter should not discharge his gun close to the entrance of the animal's hole, but should rather seek to decoy the wily reynard from his lair by means of some tempting bait, as of a fowl or sucking-pig. Listen, then, dear reader! Where a disease exists, there, too, must exist unhealthy matter. To dissolve and expel this is tantamount to luring out and capturing the fox. A douche, however, neither dissolves nor expels. When once the unhealthy matter has been removed, then light douches may render good service, and I frequently made use of them.

Itch.

This disgusting complaint may cause much havoc, both outside and inside the body.

A man, aged twenty-eight, whose appearance resembled a worm-eaten board, once came to consult me. He had failed to find help anywhere, and no one knew what was the matter with him. I asked the patient whether in his youth he had ever been afflicted with itch? He answered in the affirmative, adding that he had been cured of it within three days; but that might heaven preserve him from such another cure!

In these repulsive complaints, which more than any other denote the presence of poisonous germs in the system, the rule holds good to expel all superfluous matter from the body.

With a view to this our patient took daily for three days in succession a warm bath (106° F.) with fir-tree decoction. A thorough soaping did excellent service, by opening the pores and removing dirt. After the baths were given, complete lavations at night from bed during the first week, and a fourth warm bath terminated by a cold lavation. In the second week a warm bath with cold lavation, and a cold semi-bath with lavation of the upper body. In the third week a cold whole bath, and in future every month or two a couple of warm baths. Should the complaint prove obstinate, then the two last applications might be continued. Even one warm bath taken weekly might render good service.

In six weeks our unfortunate patient was cured, and able to select a profession. His health continues to be excellent, and the former complaint has never reappeared.

This is the treatment for suppressed itch, which has been driven from the surface to the interior.

Whoever suffers from external itch should take a warm bath (106° to 109° F.) and rub himself well with sharp soap. The so-called green soap, to be procured in any pharmacy, is best. After a quarter of an hour let him wash himself over with clean water (hot or cold) and common soap. The most effective plan would be for the patient to take a second warm bath on the back of the first, terminated by warm or cold lavation.

As itch may often be conveyed by articles of clothing, linen, &c., great care must be taken thoroughly to change all clothes, bed and body linen, &c., after the bath. If this is not done, all applications will be in vain.

In three to four days, itch may be cured in this fashion.

Jaundice.

The gall-bladder is situated in the liver, and from thence the gall flows into two canals. In these canals there sometimes form indurations proceeding from the liver, and called gall-stones. These may occasion obstruction in the flow of gall; but sometimes an accident, such as a blow or pressure, may divert some portion of gall from its proper canal and cause it to mix with the blood. This is the origin of jaundice, which also frequently follows after a severe illness, such as typhus fever, &c. Sometimes, again, the liver itself is affected, and the blood in consequence is diseased and gradually poisoned. If jaundice be produced by any accident, or should be the result of a foregoing illness, it is usually of small importance; but if it be derived from a liver complaint, it will not unfrequently prove fatal. The first signs of jaundice are to be seen in the white of the eye, then in the skin, in the stools and urine. The appetite is mostly impaired, and the taste vitiated.

If the liver be sound, then the complaint will not be difficult to heal. As internal medicine I particularly recommend three or four spoonfuls of wormwood-tea, taken three or four times daily, or else a pinch of wormwood-powder in six to ten spoonfuls of hot water. A tea made of sage and wormwood mixed will render excellent service.

Six peppercorns swallowed daily with the food, is likewise a good means of promoting digestion. Sobriety in eating and drinking is much to be recommended. Milk is an excellent nourishment in this disease.

The best water applications are: two or three times weekly a short swathing, and a complete lavation at night taken from bed. The yellow colour often remains fixed for several weeks, but is by no means dangerous. As a stuff cannot be bleached all at once of its colour, so it is with jaundice. If, however, the yellow hue becomes intensified, and gradually deepens to brown or even black, if the appetite steadily decrease, if there be a universal burning and itching throughout the skin, and if the emaciation be on the increase, then it is much to be apprehended that the liver is fatally attacked, and that induration or cancer of the liver may have set in.

Kidneys, Disease of the.

A peasant related: "I am as wretched as I appear to be strong and stout. I cannot work, am always inflated, and the difficulty in breathing is often so great that I dread suffocation. In bed I toss from side to side without being able to sleep. My urine is mostly thick and mixed with blood. I have frequently a violent sense of burning in the bladder. I have had various doctors. One of these said that I was suffering from a liver complaint and had gall-stones. A second one declared it to be a distension of the kidneys. A third one found the seat of the illness in the stomach!"

The following applications were prescribed to the almost despairing man:—

1. In the week, two warm baths of boiled oat-straw decoction (100° to 104° F.), with threefold transition into cold water (ten minutes in the warm, one minute in the cold water).

2. Two short swathings weekly, likewise dipped in oat-straw decoction, one and a half hour.

3. Daily two cupfuls of shave-grass tea with juniper-berries, boiled for ten minutes.

In six weeks the man was perfectly cured. His body is normal, the large belly disappeared, the brown-yellow complexion has given place to a healthy colour; he has likewise regained his former strength.

Knee, Inflamed.

A woman, thirty years old, had a violent inflammation from the ankle to above the knee. The swelling was sometimes very painful, quite hard and hot. The patient employed various remedies during half a year, amongst others a bandage of plaster of Paris for twelve weeks, and a second one for eight weeks. The condition was so aggravated that she could no longer put her foot to the ground, the knee in particular being acutely painful. As everything had been attempted in vain, she made a trial with infused hot hay-flowers bandaged over from the ankle to the middle of the thigh. The pains soon ceased, and when the swelling was reduced by one-half, affusions were applied to the suffering limb every second day. After eight weeks the woman began to use her leg again, and was soon able to resume her hard work.

Lungs, Emphysema.

It frequently happens that people in the prime of life suffer from difficulty in breathing, and have sometimes the painful and alarming sensation of being about to be suffocated.

Such persons are often tolerably corpulent, and of habits calculated to increase the evil. The principal cause of the complaint is usually a general weakness of the system, which is mostly languid, indolent, and bloodless. I would compare such persons to a machine whose individual parts are intact; but whose strength is not adapted to the work it has to perform. Further causes of the complaint are almost invariably unhealthy gases, which, forming in the abdomen, exercise a pressure upon the upper organs. The first step towards removing the complaint will be to expel these noxious gases, the second to brace and harden the system, and strengthen it by means of a simple nourishing diet. My thirty years' experience has taught me that this complaint may, if neglected, turn to Bright's disease.

A gentleman, under forty and tolerably stout, used occasionally to have such violent suffocating fits that he lived in apprehension of not surviving one or two more such attacks. His doctor was of the same opinion. The lack of breath was so great that the sounds produced by the patient in breathing were heard through the ceiling in the lower storey of the house. These attacks of breathlessness were tolerably lengthy, and used to leave the patient perfectly weak and exhausted. After he had rallied, he felt quite strong and healthy. Sometimes the attacks were suspended for several days, only to return again with renewed violence.

This gentleman had a strong aversion to cold water, and could only be persuaded to have recourse to it when all other means had failed. For six weeks he made use of various applications. The cure was so complete that the attacks never returned, and the gentleman has since—it is now sixteen years ago—been in full enjoyment of excellent health.

For several days the patient took a tea which had the effect of promoting profuse but painless stools: he then made use of the short swathing, upper and lower compress, and finally of the semi and complete bath, each for the space of one minute. The Spanish mantle likewise did good service. The applications were most efficacious when employed in the following order:—

First, the short swathing, which began to expel the gases and to remove and dissolve their causes; then the upper and lower compress, a continuation of the first application, which likewise tends to strengthen the system; furthermore, the Spanish mantle—this draws out the latent matter through the skin; finally, semi-baths, to brace the system.

A priest had suffered from severe inflammation of the lungs, which had left emphysema behind it, and a violent cough inexpressibly painful to hear. His appearance indicated suffering; the appetite poor, and the strength diminishing. The lungs might still be cured, the doctors declared.

The applications employed during fourteen days were as follows:—

1. Every day two upper affusions.
2. Walking in water, twice daily from three to five minutes.
3. A shawl thrice weekly.
4. Every second day a sitz-bath of one minute.

As internal medicine the patient was to take a decoction of fenugreek boiled with honey, a spoonful every hour.

The effect of the affusions was to strengthen the whole upper body. At first the cough grew stronger, and much glutinous matter was discharged. After three days, cough and expectoration diminished, and in twelve days only a very little glutinous matter remained. This was finally entirely removed by the further applications of upper affusion, knee affusion, and tea of nettle and ribwort. After three weeks the cure was complete.

LUNGS, INFLAMMATION OF.

Margaretha is lying in bed. She has a racking dry cough, accompanied by nausea, and the heat increases hourly. She feels a burning stabbing pain in the chest, and at one side. The doctor declares inflammation of the lungs to be impending. How can the patient be relieved? Every child is aware that a sponge is capable of absorbing and retaining much water. Are there no means existing by which, as water is absorbed by a sponge, so the heat may be extracted from the body? Yes, there are such means, and they lie close at hand. Every peasant-woman in our country knows the *Topfenkäs*, made out of curdled milk.[1] This cheese, together with a little of the whey, is rubbed to a fine paste, spread upon linen, and applied to the affected spot, from whence the heat and inflammation threaten to spread. I know of no other remedy which has such power to extract the heat. I have seen the greatest heats arrested and extinguished by this means, if daily repeated from two to four times, according to necessity. I am acquainted with many persons who owe their life to this simple remedy.

To still the internal heat, the patient should swallow twice daily a spoonful of olive-oil.

Should these two remedies prove ineffectual, and the heat still continue unabated, then water applications may be resorted to. The patient's whole body up to the armpits should be wrapped in a wet sheet (lower swathing), and this repeated twice daily. Or else

[1] Curdled milk is placed upon the warm hearth. It resolves itself into a thick and watery substance. The liquid part is the *topfen* water, the firm substance is known by the name of *Topfenkäs*.

the feet can be swathed above the ankle in cloths dipped in vinegar-and-water, and these renewed as often as they have become warm. The cloths may be replaced by wet socks, with dry ones drawn over them.

If the sick Margaretha makes use of this plaster during three to five days, from the very beginning of the illness, she can be completely cured within six to seven, or at the longest nine to ten days.

Other parts of the body may be attacked by inflammation as well as the lungs. We speak of inflammation of the chest, diaphragm, abdomen, &c. To all of these apply the same treatment as given above —viz., arrest and divert the conflux of blood, and extract the heat from the affected spot by the influence of cold.

I was once called at midnight to a sick man. He could hardly breathe. Cough and retching were very great. In the chest, especially at one side, he had the sensation of being stabbed by knives. I did not prepare him for death, as his relatives requested me to do, but caused him instead to be wrapped up to the armpits in wet linen cloths (lower swathing), and applied a cheese-plaster to the painful spot. That relieved him. This treatment was continued for six days, and the patient was out of danger.

Migraine, or Megrim.

Migraine (or megrim), or the semi-headache, is a peculiarly feminine complaint, which, however, is often shared by the strongest men, especially such as are addicted to much severe mental labour. Many a one has been reassured by the doctor's verdict, "Do not be alarmed; no fool ever gets a migraine." This complaint is often caused by imperfect circulation, more frequently still by disturbing influences proceeding from the stomach and abdomen.

Migraine often follows in the train of severe illness, when nature has not yet completely recovered, nor the organs regained their normal action. Migraine may also be hereditary.

This headache is easy to cure. If it proceed from unhealthy gases, it will mostly suffice vigorously to rub the abdomen with very cold water two to four times a-day for two or three days in succession. Not only are the gases often expelled by this simple process, but it acts directly on the stools, and not infrequently restores complete order. The effect will be still stronger if some vinegar or salt be mixed with the water.

Should these applications not prove strong enough, then two or three semi-baths may be taken within a week. These ought to suffice. The patient may simultaneously take some tea calculated to destroy or expel the gases. Caraway or fennel, prepared as tea, has an excellent effect. Other little household remedies are not to be despised. Five drops of lavender-oil upon sugar will render the same service. Many have obtained relief from six to eight juniper-berries, taken at intervals during the day.

Nervous Complaint.

A priest related as follows:—

"In consequence of great excitement, anxiety, and fright, I got a complaint towards the end of July 1884, which declared itself by frequent palpitations of the heart, shortness of breath, and general weakness. The palpitations ceased after some months; but in exchange I got other complaints—violent attacks of asthma, and frequent painful pressure in the neighbourhood of the ribs, and sometimes in the spinal marrow. I often experience the greatest weakness and weariness in all my limbs, and pain in the joints. Constipation and flatulency also trouble me. My voice is so much weakened that simple speaking occasions breathlessness and asthma, and it is quite impossible to use the voice consecutively for any length of time. During the whole time I am afflicted with pressure on the head, dizziness, sometimes violent headache, so that I am scarcely able to think, and am quite incapable of any mental work. Every trifle excites me, and greatly increases the pressure on the chest and head. Deep melancholy has attacked my spirit, and I sometimes almost despair. The doctors declare my malady to be a nervous complaint. Two of these, an allopathist and a homœopathist, both celebrated men, prescribed various remedies (douche-baths, diet, bromkali, Zincum oxydæ, Natron. phosph., &c.), which all failed to cure, and rather increased the complaint. The only relief afforded to me was by cold baths and much exercise in the fresh air, which a third doctor advised. This lasted for half a year, till at last I took refuge in cold water."

In appearance this patient was unusually red, the eyeballs somewhat yellow, lips and ears deep red mixed with blue. The young man's hair (he was scarcely above thirty) had almost entirely fallen out. All these symptoms pointed to an unusual conflux of blood towards head and chest. The pains in the forehead denote the rush of blood to the head, whereby the veins are distended. A cure can only be effected by diverting the blood towards the extremities; then only can I proceed to dissolve whatever be superfluous (agglomerations, distension of veins, &c.) in head and chest, and finally act upon the whole system.

The best applications are these, taken in the following order: vapour foot-bath, vapour head-bath, short swathing, Spanish mantle, walking on stones, upper and lower affusion, Spanish mantle, walking barefoot, (in new-fallen snow if it be winter-time).

Within three weeks the condition was much improved, but months were required in order completely to cure such an inrooted and advanced complaint.

Nervous Exhaustion.

A pastor related that he was sometimes a prey to intolerable headache, and that whenever this relaxed, he got such oppression in the throat as hardly to be able to speak for pain and fatigue. Also in the back he suffered from frequent weariness and painful spasms. The doctor's certificate, which he brought, declared him to be suffering from complete nervous exhaustion, which threatened to attack the brain and spine. Extreme irritation and a sense of anxiety were likewise present.

Applications: daily a weak upper affusion, morning and afternoon; walking once daily in wet grass and on wet stones, for four minutes. So on for five days. After that, daily a stronger upper affusion, a knee affusion, and walking twice in water. Thus also for five days more, with sitz-baths between times.

The further applications were: daily a back affusion,

a semi-bath, an upper affusion, and walking in water. These applications removed all sufferings; happy and healthy the patient returned to the duties of his vocation.

Nervous Surexcitation.

Two students came to me during the Easter holidays, and related: "We suffer from headache, determination of blood to the head, impaired sleep and appetite, and great weariness. We are incapable of thus continuing. Cannot we make use of the holidays in order to regain our health by the cold-water cure?"

As it was spring-time, and the ground still moist and tolerably cold, I gave them the advice to spend their holidays in walking barefoot in the woods and meadows, with rapid exercise whenever they felt cold; also from time to time to stand or walk about from two to three minutes in a stream or ditch filled with water.

In like manner they were told to put their arms completely in water two or three times daily. The young people found these applications very congenial; spirits and courage revived; with renewed zest they returned to their studies, were able to perform their tasks with ease, and joyfully looked forward to the autumn vacation in order to resume the work of bracing their system.

A similar case was that of a seminarist, who came to me with the following lamentations: "I have such violent pressure on the head that I sometimes scarcely know where I am and what I am doing. I frequently suffer from dizziness, am incapable of mental work, and was obliged to leave the college three months before the term."

It was in warm August weather, and this student

spent ten days in the garden and woods walking barefoot from morning to evening. In addition he daily received from two to four upper affusions. In twelve days the symptoms of his complaint had disappeared; he felt cheerful and strengthened, and in order to regain complete health, he merely required thus to spend the rest of his vacation time.

PALSY.

A pastor was stricken down by palsy. One hand, one foot, and all one side were completely lamed, speech and consciousness arrested. All medical remedies were tried for several days without effect. The doctor finally declared that one side was completely paralysed, and would remain so, and that in all probability a second stroke would soon come to lame the other side and put an end to his life. A trial with water, thought I, can therefore do no harm. No sooner said than done! The cold leg and arm were vigorously washed with cold water on the first day; two warm foot-baths, with vigorous lavation of the feet, and four lavations of the upper body, were the applications of the second day. Already on the third day it was perceived that in the two paralysed limbs life and sensibility still existed. This encouraged me. On the fourth day we managed with difficulty to apply a lower swathing to the helpless body for one hour, and placed the semi-lifeless feet twice in a warm foot-bath with salt and ashes. This was continued for fourteen days. At the end of this time the patient was able to assist us in the process with his healthy hand and foot, and he joyfully showed that he was now able slightly to raise the paralysed hand. Complete lavations were now applied daily, and once weekly a head or foot vapour-bath—alternate weeks. So on for three weeks. Renewed vigour began to pervade the shattered tree, the appetite increased, and each of the three following weeks was filled up with one warm bath (with transition into cold), one vapour head-bath, one vapour foot-bath, and three semi-baths, with lavation of the upper body (for one minute). The conclusion of the cure consisted in upper and lower affusions, alternated with the Spanish mantle. The work was long, tedious, and fatiguing; but the old gentleman recovered so far as to be able daily to say Mass again, to visit the sick, hold all services, and accomplish all necessary writing. The only thing he never recovered was the power to preach. The tongue had suffered too much, and there were some words which he could only pronounce with difficulty.

The stroke here described took place about ten years ago. The gentleman is still alive and in good health.

A man, forty-five years old, had a stroke of apoplexy. His right hand and foot were quite insensible, the appetite completely awanting. The patient's upper body and feet were daily washed with a mixture of vinegar and warm water. Thrice daily he took thirty drops of wormwood, sage, and marsh-clover. By the end of a fortnight hands and feet had regained their habitual warmth and sensation, and the man was able to walk about the room. The appetite increased, the paralysed side gradually regained strength, and in a few days the whole system was restored to order.

A general remark here may be of use to many. Should any one be attacked with palsy, and partial paralysis have set in, let vigorous cold lavations be immediately applied to the patient's back, chest, and abdomen, from two to four times daily. Salt or vinegar may be mixed with the water. In like manner legs and arms should be washed over, in order to promote uniform circulation. All these applications should be performed as rapidly as possible, none lasting above one minute.

If the paralysis be trifling, and the patient able to sit upright, a vapour head-bath of twenty minutes' duration, with subsequent cold lavation, should be first applied. Four to six hours later may follow a vapour foot-bath, likewise for twenty minutes, concluded by a cold lavation or knee affusion. The other aforementioned applications may then be pursued.

Complete swathings are to be avoided in the beginning, nature being still too weak to replace the latent heat thus withdrawn. I know a case in which the doctor wished to cure a patient by means of complete swathings. The first application appeared to improve his condition; but after the second swathing the patient remained cold, and his body had assumed a bluish colour. Only by the application of heat was he again brought round to life.

PERSPIRATION.

Many people are afflicted with continual violent sweating of the feet, combined with a foul smell. This is very disagreeable, but it would be a great mistake to seek to suppress this perspiration by violent measures. Who wishes to catch a fox will never be so foolish as to stop up the mouth of his hole.

Perspiration of the feet is in reality nothing else but foul indolent secretions, which infect and corrupt the vessels containing them.

The surest and most effectual manner of curing this complaint is to wrap both feet in cloths dipped in hay-flower or pine-tree decoction.

These compresses will draw out the unhealthy matter, and both plants have the same healing and strengthening virtues. Five or six of these swathings should be employed for ten days. During the next fourteen days, a warm foot-bath reaching to the calves for ten minutes daily, and with three transitions, of one minute each, into cold water. Finally, one of the aforementioned swathings and one foot-bath in the week. After the complaint has been removed, it will be good to walk barefoot from time to time a quarter of an hour in wet grass. Those who cannot do this may walk barefoot about their room for a few minutes before bed-time. No one would believe how salutary, refreshing, invigorating, and bracing is this simple practice.

Besides foot-sweating, there may also exist a general unhealthy sweating of the whole person, attended by a foul smell.

A gentleman of distinction used to perspire so profusely that every morning his whole mattress, sheets, and pillows were dripping wet. He suffered, moreover, from almost continual catarrhs.

No one should attempt to cure this complaint suddenly. The course of applications pursued by the aforesaid gentleman, and crowned with complete success, were as follows:—

Thrice weekly a Spanish mantle for one and a half to two hours. Twice to thrice weekly (either in the day or night time) a complete lavation taken from bed. As further applications, after the complaint has ceased, one complete lavation in the week will do no harm.

There are also persons afflicted by excessive, though not offensive, sweating, called forth by the slightest exertion, which occasions much weariness, and renders the subjects liable to colds, catarrhs, inflammation, &c.

An official who came to visit me one day suffered from this complaint, combined with bad digestion and difficulty in breathing. I gave him the advice to take a cold semi-bath, with lavation of the upper body, whenever he returned home bathed in perspiration. The whole proceeding should not last more than one minute, after which he was to dress again and take exercise for a quarter of an hour in his room. The gentleman first thought I was merely joking, and could with difficulty be persuaded to follow my advice, which ran so contrary to his preconceived ideas. A fortnight later he thanked me warmly for having relieved this disagreeable complaint. He is still alive, and not far short of eighty years.

A last remark must here find place. Few things are more dreaded by the majority of people than the contact of cold when they are in perspiration. This preconceived notion may have arisen from the fact that many persons have caught cold from the effects of a cold draught upon their perspiring bodies. My experience, however, has taught me to hold by the following rules:—

(*a*) Whoever is wet through perspiration, rain, &c., should avoid cold air or draught.

(*b*) Whoever shivers should never attempt a cold-water application.

(*c*) Whoever has been drenched by rain, should change his clothes as fast as possible.

(*d*) But he who perspires—whether this be owing to a diseased state of the system, or the result of heat, exercise, work, &c.—may fearlessly indulge in a rapid cold bath or complete lavation, if he be careful to resume his clothes quickly without drying, and take exercise until the body be completely dry, and have regained its normal temperature.

PILES.

Piles may either be hereditary or else acquired from a sedentary or over-indulgent mode of life. The simple countryman who goes about his daily work, and nourishes himself on milk and potatoes, hardly ever knows this complaint, even by name.

Piles are very troublesome and painful, though seldom a dangerous malady. Not only do they cause much itching and burning, but likewise react upon the mind, inducing despondency and low spirits, which sometimes lead to the verge of insanity.

But what are piles, and how are they formed? Every one has seen how the turkey-cock's fleshy neck sometimes hangs down limply like empty sacks. But let something arouse his ire, and straightway these sacks will be filled with blood like little red balls. In like manner piles are nothing else but little sacks filled with blood or slimy matter.

Veins are elastic tubes. Whenever there is an irregular conflux of blood towards any particular spot, there the dammed-up blood forms stagnant pools. Thus originate on hands and face little wart-like knots, which are filled with blood. When these take place inside the rectum, they are called invisible piles; visible piles are those which protrude outwardly.

From time to time these bags break open and discharge their contents, sometimes a brown slimy matter, often, however, pure blood. The patient always feels relieved after these discharges. Not only in the rectum are these parasites to be found, in degenerate systems they are likewise formed in the interior of the body, and inside the principal arteries.

The more numerous these knots, and the more frequently they break open, the greater injury is occasioned to the spot where they congregate. Incurable sores and ulcers, cancer of the rectum, &c., are the not infrequent result.

This complaint is sometimes aggravated by the ascarides (little worms) which penetrate into the rectum, and there easily occasion malignant tumours.

The treatment of piles with water is easy and mostly successful. The number of those to whom I have brought relief is very great, and I may add that all cases were brought to a successful conclusion.

Let us first attack the ascarides, if these pernicious leeches be present. Their presence is mostly betrayed by a sense of itching and burning in the rectum (though this may likewise be occasioned by the piles themselves, when refilling with blood). Take one, two, or three cold-water injections in rapid succession, and allow these to flow off again at once. When the cold water enters the rectum it usually dislodges the ascarides, like leeches when strewn over with salt. If this be repeated two or three times (it may take place twice or thrice weekly) a great many, sometimes all, of the tiny tormentors will be removed.

The following remarks apply to those cases in which we have to do with simple piles only. Wherever there is an excessive conflux of blood, it must be diverted and dispersed; vessels which have been unduly distended should be contracted, impurities and unhealthy matter are to be removed.

For all these conditions the following application is good: Prepare a lower compress in bed, long enough to reach from the nape of the neck to over the rectum. The patient lies down upon this for three-quarters of an hour, repeating the process from three to four times weekly. Should the compress absorb much heat before the three-quarters of an hour have elapsed, then it should be removed and renewed.

As further applications, three or four sitz-baths weekly will be found useful, if taken cold and rapid. These can also be taken at night straight from bed, never longer than from one to two minutes.

Sufferers from chronic piles should try this mode of treatment for one or two weeks every three months: if it fail entirely to remove the complaint, it will at least prevent it from acquiring serious dimensions.

Bran bread (of which the recipe is given in the second part of this work) is much to be recommended to those who suffer from piles. Many persons have assured me that since using it in their daily diet they have experienced much relief, as it serves, if not wholly to cure the complaint, at least to keep it in check.

Respiration, Difficult.

A priest related as follows: "I am well built, was always healthy and vigorous, but for three-quarters of a year I have suffered so much from gathering and phlegm that I often feel in danger of suffocation. I used to have a strong sonorous voice, but now I can hardly render myself intelligible; likewise I am often so weary that I can scarce drag myself along. Various doctors have pronounced it to be respectively chest or bronchial catarrh."

Applications—

From three to four times daily an upper affusion, and twice a-day walking in water which reaches over the calves. This course to be continued for four days. After the first four days, two upper affusions daily, one back affusion, and a semi-bath. In addition to this, walking daily in water. This second treatment will occupy five more days, after which daily, one semi-bath, one back affusion, one upper affusion, and one knee affusion.

The whole cure was soon accomplished, and immense quantities of phlegm withdrawn from the patient. Day by day his looks improved; the breathing became easier, the voice clearer, the humour more cheerful. The complaint had originally been caused by want of exercise and over-warm clothing.

Rheumatism.

Innumerable persons are tormented by rheumatism in head, feet, arms, legs, back, or chest.

The hard-working peasant, the wood-cleaver, and all those engaged in hard active labour, know little of this illness, because, in my opinion, these people often catch rheumatism in one hour to lose it again in the next. They may, for instance, be attacked by rheumatic pains in the morning, and have worked them off again the same afternoon.

This last observation gives us a clear hint how to cure rheumatism. When rheumatism is deep-seated, contrary to my usual habit, I summon friction to assist the action of water. By this means heat is more rapidly produced, and the chief cause of the complaint more quickly dispelled. If the affected parts, being cold, were to be immediately affused with cold water without previous warming, the rheumatism would thereby but be made to retreat further into the body.

A veterinary surgeon once lamented to me his incapability further to pursue his profession on account of the dreadful rheumatism, which, like a vicious cat, had dug its claws into his right shoulder. He had taken cold from going out inadvertently when bathed in perspiration; and he felt convinced that, as had happened several times, he would have to carry this troublesome cat about with him fully six weeks.

"If you wish, sir," I answered him, "in twenty-four hours you will be delivered of your complaint. I shall set on my dog to chase away your cat." He laughed, and we made a bet on the subject.

I bade him go home, cause his back to be first vigorously rubbed dry by his wife, and then apply a cold upper affusion. Eight hours later he took a vapour head-bath, with subsequent cold affusion. The twenty-four hours had not yet struck before the cat had taken French leave, and I had won my bet.

A peasant got such violent rheumatic pains in both

legs that he could not walk any more. The thighs in particular were greatly pained. He did not know how he had caught the complaint.

This peasant daily wrapped himself in a lower swathing, dipped in hot hay-flower decoction, and reaching to the armpits, and laid himself each time in bed, for two hours, well covered up. Ten such applications sufficed completely to cure the rheumatism.

Another peasant could not endure the swathing because of the violent pains in the legs. He was put into an oat-straw bath, 106° to 111° F., twice daily for twenty-five minutes, each time with threefold transition into the cold. In three days he was cured.

Cases of rheumatism in the head I could relate in plenty. They were usually cured by doing little or nothing to the head itself, but directing warm baths and vapour applications to the legs. The best sequence of applications is the following:—

A warm foot-bath, with salt and ashes.
A shawl.
A vapour foot-bath.
A head vapour-bath.
A shawl.

One of these applications daily will cure the most violent head rheumatism.

No rheumatism should be neglected, as it may lay the seeds of manifold severe diseases of lungs, ears, eyes, &c., as also of inflammation, blood-poisoning, ulcers, &c.

A gentleman comes: his appearance is sickly, and his expression one of deep melancholy and suffering. At once the thought occurred to me, This man is suffering, or has suffered much. The complexion is of an unwholesome yellow hue, his hair is very scarce. His own account of his state was as follows: "I have frequently suffered from violent fits of colic and diarrhœa, with much pain. Later I got a disease of the kidneys, as the doctors called it. When the terrible pains took hold of me, they turned me round like a spindle or a whipping-top. After years I lost this complaint, but I got instead this acute rheumatism. It seems to me as if all former pains had now assumed this form, in order to torture each separate joint. I have tried many medical remedies, none of which procured the desired result, but left me with the old pains. With great difficulty, and by dint of much self-command, I have continued to fulfil my duties till now. I never complained to any one, for no one understood me, not even the doctor. He who has promised a crown to those who suffer, alone knows what my sufferings have been. I must still mention one thing. My feet used to be affected by a dry perspiration: the remedies I was advised to use cured this, but I have not felt well since then. I have also taken mineral baths, but they only increased my complaint."

What may be the root of all these complaints? The question is not difficult to answer. The patient's own words have given us the clue, and we only require to draw the conclusion. His yellow complexion, the frequent attacks of colic, the suppressed foot-perspiration, all point to some poisonous matter which, like a snake in the grass, lurks in the body, sometimes hissing and putting out its forked tongue, till now, with a last attack it seizes on its prey with poisonous fangs, sending the venom throughout the body into the very blood and marrow. Also, the hair does not fall from the scalp of a healthy person without special cause. An internal storm must be here at work, shaking off the hair as the wind in autumn carries off the sear and withered leaves.

Cure can only be effected when this poisonous matter, which has corroded everything, is dissolved and expelled from the body. My patient was first ordered to take the Spanish mantle. This was succeeded by a head vapour-bath, followed by a vigorous cold lavation, and then a foot vapour-bath. Between these two vapour applications, a tolerable interval always took place; for the more carefully and leniently the body is treated, the easier will it be for the patient to endure the applications, and for nature to assist the process. After this the patient received a short swathing, and, by way of invigorating the system, an upper and lower affusion. Of each of the aforementioned applications one daily; besides this, every night from bed a complete lavation. In the fourth and fifth weeks he received weekly two semi-baths, one head vapour-bath, one foot vapour-bath, and one Spanish mantle; finally, in the sixth week, two warm baths alternated with cold, one semi-bath, and one upper and lower affusion. For future treatment I recommended the patient to employ one or two complete lavations weekly, an upper and a lower affusion, and once a-month a warm bath, without transition into cold.

Water did not belie my anticipations even in this complicated case. The grave complaint, which doubtless would have resulted in death, disappeared. Lost strength returned, with a fresh healthy complexion, and renewed courage and energy took the place of his former despondency.

A man, aged about forty, had such violent rheumatic pains in one leg that he could only walk short distances with the help of a stick. Sometimes he had also pains in the arms and shoulders. He had tried various remedies without avail. At last he had recourse to water, and in six days had almost shaken off the complaint; he continued the applications, and was completely cured.

The applications were as follows:—

During six days two upper affusions daily, and two lower affusions; once in the week a swathing under the arms; twice daily walking in water reaching above the calves, from one to three minutes. Every day a back affusion and walking in wet grass.

Ringworm of the Scalp.

A peasant's daughter related: "For two years I have suffered from a permanent eruption on the head and face, which is sometimes stronger, sometimes weaker. Under the hair there form many little fistules, from which a sharp liquid comes. My body itches frequently, and I feel much internal heat. I have taken many medicines, especially purgatives, but am not cured.

"Cold-water cure completely restored me within six weeks. I took the following applications:—

"1. In the week thrice from bed a complete lavation, returning to bed at once.

"2. Every week a wet shirt dipped in salt water.

"3. A vapour head-bath once in the week.

"4. Once in the week a wet shirt, and once or twice a complete lavation.

"As medicine, twenty drops of juniper extract in a glass of water twice daily."

Rupture.

This complaint has nowadays become frequent, and often appears overnight like toadstools in the forest; sometimes, however, it is preceded by pains at particular spots. All thus attacked are henceforth unfit for violent exertion, and the least imprudence in this respect may be attended with danger or even death.

Rupture is of most frequent occurrence in weak constitutions, and is often to be met with in these days of effeminacy and enervation. I am fully convinced that were our youth to be rationally brought up and hardened, such complaints would be almost unknown, unless when accidentally caused by some violent outer influence, as a blow or push.

Fifty years ago there were very few such "broken people" to be met with in a village; in the town they could be counted on the fingers. Nowadays, among twenty, three or four will be found to be thus affected. The patient usually tries to conceal his complaint, not liking to confess that he has a rupture. This false shame prevents many from seeking rational help and advice, and thus the small evil grows into a large one. Rupture is not only to be found amongst those who toil laboriously for their daily bread; it also occurs not infrequently among the higher classes. How quickly it may be brought about! Such a one jumped over a ditch and got rupture; while in such another it was caused by accumulation of gas in the abdomen. A third case, again, was that of a priest who, having delivered a sermon with much vehemence, received his rupture in the pulpit.

With few exceptions rupture is not an innate or hereditary complaint, but has been caused by weakness, either constitutional or acquired. Had the system been properly braced and hardened, especially by judicious cold-water applications, this might easily have been prevented or cured. Will the so-called civilised world ever become wise? I doubt it. But thou, honest hard-working countryman, who readest these lines, follow my advice and take once or twice in the week a cold semi-bath or sitz-bath (any tub may be made to serve the purpose). Its invigorating effects will soon be felt. Any time in the day is suitable for the purpose, and the whole proceeding, with dressing and undressing, should not occupy above four to six minutes at the outside. Take it straight away from thy work, and be not deterred because of thy profuse perspiration. Never fear! It will do thee no harm. Sit down in the water up to the chest, and quickly wash over the upper body, then dress again and back to work.

A peasant once complained to me of strong pains in the groins. The doctor was of opinion that a rupture was about to appear. I advised him diligently to employ upper and lower compresses. Soon the pains decreased. The peasant suspended his hard labour for a short time, and so escaped the anticipated complaint. Made wise by the warning he had received, he became henceforth an ardent cold-water disciple.

Finally, still the question, Can rupture, when once formed, never be cured?

Cases of recent rupture, even in adults, I have frequently cured by rubbing the spot with camphor-oil, and then applying a plaster made of pitch spread upon linen. Fox's grease was, and is still, one of the most efficient remedies for new ruptures. Rub with it the affected spot for two or three days successively, and apply the pitch-plaster as above. In this manner I once cured a rupture that was over nine weeks old.

Children are often subject to rupture. The usual cause is, that their bodies being unnaturally distended by food, the intestines get easily displaced and burst the peritoneum. Let the child thus affected take daily an oat-straw bath, and likewise daily an upper and lower compress, until the cure be complete. The spot may also be rubbed with camphor-oil, or, better still, fox's grease. These damages usually heal quickly, unless they have already assumed large dimensions, in which case a complete cure is hardly possible.

In such cases the patient's only resource will be a truss, which must be worn according to surgical directions.

Mothers who truly love their children should be attentive to avert and counteract this complaint whenever its first symptoms appear. Much may depend upon this, as it involves the child's whole future life and health, and the parents' consequent happiness or misery.

Saint Vitus's Dance.

A father related: "I have a daughter, now ten years old, who, since her infancy, has never been healthy. She suffered so much in teething that we thought she would die. Moreover, one leg became thinner than the other. Now the girl has got St

Vitus's dance; she can neither eat nor sleep, and it is dreadful to witness when the cramps befall her. I have sought help from many doctors, but her condition gets ever worse."

"Good man, boil aftermath for half an hour with water—take plenty, in order that the water may be thick—put in some salt, and dip a coarse shirt in the water; wring it well out and put on the child; then wrap the child in a warm blanket, and let her lie thus for one and a half to two hours: if she sleep, do not rouse her, even should the two hours have elapsed. Do so for eight days, twice daily, then come and bring me news."

After eight days the man returned and said: "The girl has got a terrible eruption on the whole body, especially upon chest and back; the cramps have ceased; she sleeps well, and has a good appetite. What shall I now do further?"

Answer: "Give the child the wet shirt as before, every third day, and when this has been done for fourteen days, the child will be cured. Give her also every day about twenty of these wormwood drops in water as hitherto."

Scarlet Fever.

An epidemic of scarlet fever mostly breaks out once or twice in every year, and carries off numerous victims. It usually attacks children, though adults too are not always spared. The foreboding symptoms of this disease are headache, pressure on the stomach and chest, languor, and alternating heat and cold. Though very fatal to children, scarlet fever may easily be subdued by means of cold water. Children are usually out of danger at the end of two days;

with adults the recovery is somewhat slower. Scarlet fever can readily be cured in the following manner: Should a child (no matter its age) be attacked with the symptoms of the complaint, dip a shirt in hot salt water, wring out thoroughly, and put on the patient, who must be brought to bed and well covered up. At the end of an hour remove the shirt, and the child's skin will be found profusely covered with the scarlet eruption. Should the heat continue to be great, a rapid complete lavation may be applied. In serious cases, when the heat goes on increasing and there is a sense of much anxiety, the wet shirt may be repeated two or three times in one day; sometimes, but rarely, as often as four times. Everything depends upon the heat and strength of the fever. If these decrease, then the intervals of time between two shirts may be proportionately increased. These later applications are to be performed with cold water mixed with vinegar. After removing the wet shirt, dress the child again in a clean linen one. Thus treated, scarlet fever can be cured in four, or, at the utmost, six days.

One remark is important. When the patient feels little or no appetite, food should on no account be pressed upon him. There is usually much thirst, for which water will always remain the best palliative. A little sugar or a few drops of wine may be mixed with the water. Country children usually prefer milk. In general, observe the rule to drink often but always in small portions, and I do not think that a child thus treated will die.

Louis, a boy of ten years, has such violent heat that he can hardly speak. His face is red, and he complains that everything hurts him. The heat and anxiety being so great, Louis is washed over with cold water every hour for two days. On the third day the boy can already begin to eat, and the lavations are reduced to twice in the course of the day. On the fifth day Louis feels quite well; on the sixth he is able to walk about the room, and very soon he has rejoined his comrades out of doors.

A girl, aged twenty-four, who had always enjoyed good health, was attacked by scarlet fever. The eruption continued to increase for eight days, reaching a pitch of which there are few examples in the disease. The patient herself demanded to be treated with cold water, in which she had much confidence. She was advised to wash herself over completely with water every hour. This interval was found to be too great, and the heat continuing to increase, she was regularly washed over every half-hour for more than five days. She hardly took any food, and only drank in small portions. Only after ten days' assiduous treatment with cold water the heat gave way: the eruption began partially to dry up, and had quite disappeared by the fourteenth day, when the girl was completely restored to health.

Sciatica.

An official suffered for more than three months from violent pains in the left hip, reaching to the ankle. He had tried many remedies, and was finally advised rest and warmth as the only means of cure. He therefore employed warm wrappings, and baths as hot as could be endured; only, however, with the result that the pains increased, while his strength daily diminished. He lost fully half a hundredweight, and could seldom sleep for an hour at a time.

At last he took courage to employ the remedy he most dreaded—cold water.

He daily received two to three applications:—

1. A back affusion in the forenoon.
2. In the afternoon upper affusion.

In the second day: in the morning, upper affusion; afternoon, back affusion. Every second or third day, a semi-bath; walking barefoot between times.

Immediately after the first affusion the patient was able to sleep four hours at night; in this way sleep returned, with improved appetite and a healthier appearance. At the end of four weeks the complaint was of no further importance, and in six weeks he was completely cured.

A Hungarian professor had suffered seven years from sciatica, and had visited various mineral watering-places, such as Baden, Teplitz, &c., without effect. He was cured within twenty-four days by the following applications: Every night a complete lavation; forenoon, upper affusion; afternoon, back affusion. Every second day a semi-bath; knee affusions and sitz-baths against constipation.

SLEEPLESSNESS.

A pastor suffered for nine weeks from sleeplessness. His strength daily decreased, and his mind became more and more unfit for exertion. Depression, weariness, and discouragement had replaced his former cheerful activity.

Great exertion and annoyance had excited the good gentleman, leaving him with a sense of bitter irritation.

Such a condition never fails to bring its revenge. His blood was like a hunted stag, endeavouring to flee from its pursuers in wild flight. Complete tranquillity was restored by the head vapour-bath, the Spanish mantle, upper affusions with knee affusion, vapour foot-bath, short swathing, upper and lower compress, —which course was continued for twelve days, from two to three applications being performed each day. Already on the third day the gentleman was able to sleep for three hours. He is still alive and in excellent health.

Sleeplessness may proceed from various causes, from disturbed circulation, suppressed or insufficient perspiration, flatulency, &c.

It mostly attacks those addicted to severe and prolonged mental work. I knew a gentleman whose mind took much, his body little, exercise. He would fain have dispensed with body, stomach, or legs. Such patients can with difficulty be made to understand reason; but in this particular case I succeeded in inducing him to bestow a few crumbs of nourishment on the soul's unfortunate companion—the body. He formed the habit of taking twice weekly the Spanish mantle. Sleeplessness soon left him, along with all the little complaints it brings in its train.

Another gentleman caused a tub of cold water to be placed near his bed every evening. If in half an hour or an hour he was still awake, then he washed over the whole body, and without drying returned to bed. If he woke again too soon, he would repeat the process a second and even a third time. I never heard this gentleman complain again of sleeplessness in later times.

It is often difficult to put children to sleep, or else they wake up soon again. Over-feeding is mostly the reason of this: their poor little bodies groan under the weight that has been laid upon them, and the ascending gases prevent the little heads from finding rest. If we take a wet towel and wrap it round the child's body, like a short swathing, it will soon fall asleep.

Country people often say that a warm footbath produces sleep, when over-fatigue and exertion prevents the eyes from closing. This, however, will hardly suffice for those afflicted with mental fatigue. To such sufferers, and to all those whose sleeplessness is caused by piles, flatulency, and other complaints of the abdomen, I recommend cold sitz-baths, one or two in the course of the night, and each of one or two minutes' duration.

A last cause of sleeplessness may be the unequal temperature of the body. If there be too much blood in head and chest, the extremities are mostly cold. The proper remedies for this condition have been elsewhere sufficiently indicated.

I can advise no one to employ narcotics or soporifics as a means of producing artificial sleep. I consider all such to be unnatural, and whatever is contrary to nature can never be wholesome.

Slime Fever.

If catarrh is to be compared to an infant, slime fever is the grown-up child. Slime fever is always developed from catarrh, and both may lead to innumerable diseases, as I had occasion to remark elsewhere. The cure, and consequently the application, is identical in both cases. Whoever wishes to cure catarrh easily and speedily, should go to bed and wash over chest, abdomen, and back every hour: three or four such applications in one night will nip a fresh catarrh in the bud. Should the catarrh progress—that is to say, should inflammation appear in throat, head, or chest—then the patient may be said to be suffering from slime fever, which is, in fact, nothing but a catarrh which has spread throughout the body. The spot where the catarrh has begun, be it throat, chest, or windpipe will, however, always remain the most sensitive until recovery has completely set in.

SMALLPOX.

Scarlet fever is poisonous, but smallpox is still more so, whether it be the distinct or benign form, or the confluent or malignant smallpox. The treatment is identical in both cases. It is commonly said that when the pocks do not form properly then the patient dies. It is therefore of the greatest importance to induce the eruption to come out freely and rapidly on the surface, and so prevent the poison from spreading internally.

Six persons attacked with the benign form of smallpox were cured by being completely washed over with cold water as often as the heat grew unbearable. In the beginning this lavation had to take place every hour, later every second hour, and finally from two to three times in the day. On the seventh day all six patients were completely cured. They had scarcely eaten anything, but had drunk a good deal, which will do no harm if the beverage be administered in small portions. If only all patients would observe this rule!

To drink much at a time does not serve permanently to assuage the thirst, and often increases the feeling of anxiety.

I have myself been frequently surprised to see how, by means of simple lavations, as above directed, the smallpox has been forced to the surface. The pustules make their appearance as small pointed erections, which rise above the skin like frogs on the water's surface. Have no fear in applying water; the sooner and the more regularly the lavations are performed, the faster will the pustules come out, and the more rapidly will the poison be expelled. Even before the pustules are fully formed, the poison will, so to say, have been washed away.

One further remark. Do not deprive the patient of fresh air, as used formerly to be the case in such maladies. At least a little chink of the window should always be left open.

The lavations should be so rapidly performed as not to occupy longer than a minute each time. Adults thus treated are as easily cured of smallpox as are children of scarlet fever, and will never be afflicted by those disfiguring marks which so many are doomed to carry about with them through life.

Spine.

A distinguished officer had injured a spinal vertebra when driving. The doctors declared the spine to be affected, and he was subject to violent pains, which scarcely ever left him, and reacted upon the mind with yet greater intensity. No doctor was able to give him help, although he had consulted the most celebrated physicians of the capital. On being told that cure was impossible, and that in time consumption must set in, this gentleman took refuge in cold water. Within six months he was cured, and is still in full enjoyment of excellent health, although this cure took place more than twenty years ago.

I cannot rightly recall to mind what applications were used in this particular case, but should any of my readers be afflicted with a like complaint, I would advise as follows: Thrice in the week a Spanish mantle; likewise thrice a semi-bath, with lavation of the upper body; and twice an upper and a lower affusion. This course should be pursued for several weeks. The whole system will thus be invigorated and strengthened, the disturbed vertebra will be restored to rest, and the other sympathetic affections will gradually disappear. I repeat here again that whenever one spot is affected, the entire body, the whole system, shares the pain of each individual little member.

Throw a stone into the water, and the whole surface of the pond is moved and disturbed by ever-widening circles. The stone is like the injured vertebra, which sends pain-circles throughout the body.

Spine, Curvature of.

A boy, aged sixteen, was afflicted with curvature of the spine. He was treated without result by various celebrated doctors for disease of the spinal marrow. They sent him to a hospital, where he was bandaged in divers fashions, and which he left upon crutches in a still worse plight than when he came there seventeen weeks previously. The hospital authorities had declared that nothing further could be done for him.

A benefactor presented the boy's father with a copy of 'My Water Cure,' out of which they learnt to make applications of water-and-vinegar, with such good results that at the end of a short time the boy was able to walk tolerably well with the aid of a stick. Hereupon the boy was brought to me, in the expectation that he would be completely cured. In seventeen days the whole cure was accomplished. The boy was able to walk again like any other youth of his age; not with the same strength perhaps, but yet with great assurance and without the assistance of a stick, and without pain. The treatment consisted in the following applications :—

A sort of waistcoat or vest was made of coarse linen stuff: this, dipped in oat-straw decoction, was put on at night, with a dry vest over it, and above all a woollen blanket. The wet vest remained on overnight; this was applied every second, and later every third evening. Every day the patient got two upper affusions and one knee affusion, or else walking in water and a semi-bath. The further applications were—every week two semi-baths, two upper affusions, and once a wet waistcoat.

Stomach Complaints.

Poor stomach! what sins are not saddled on thy back! After heart and nerves, thou art verily the chief scapegoat! Ask a hundred persons if they be not stomach-ailing? Very few indeed will answer with a decided negative. And yet in the most frequent cases the stomach is as innocent as a new-born babe, and as healthy as a cheerful frolicking boy. Let some examples confirm our assertion.

During a whole year Amalie has been forced to vomit almost whatever she swallows. She can retain nothing but three or four spoonfuls of lukewarm milk daily. She consulted several celebrated doctors. The apothecary at last declared that in his whole pharmacy there scarcely remained a medicine which she had not tried.

The patient was brought to me without previous warning, in a cart which stopped before my house. I could not send away the poor people. The unfortunate patient was much emaciated—her features drawn, the voice broken, a picture of woe. There was no cough, however (an important fact), only an obstinate stomach complaint, they told me, and I was begged to give her something for the stomach. I told them to be quiet, and not to abuse the stomach, which was this person's healthiest organ—the complaint was quite elsewhere. Some of the people were angry, and others laughed; the sick person herself was startled, and looked at me doubtfully, as though she questioned my sanity. To have come so far, and in such pain, only to hear this hard and pitiless verdict of a priest! But I cared little.

What led me to this conclusion?

The patient did not cough, but expelled much air (gases) through the mouth. Stomach and abdomen were greatly inflated with gases. In this condition no one can exist, and even the usually patient stomach was forced in great measure to relinquish its functions. The complaint was aggravated by the dryness of the skin and lack of perspiration.

The applications were prescribed in the following sequence: Lukewarm lower swathing; lavation of the upper body; short swathing; complete lavation; knee affusion (half a minute); again lower swathing; upper affusion; kneeling in water (half a minute) up to the pit of the stomach; complete lavation; upper and lower compress. Every half-day the patient had to take one of these applications in the aforenamed order, walking, besides, several times daily on wet stones.

By means of lukewarm swathings, I first thought to make the skin softer, moister, and warmer, and by the complete lavations and other applications, to act directly on the lower body. In this I succeeded; the air and gases found the proper outlet, the perspiration and normal action of the skin returned. With the disappearance of the gases, appetite awoke within the now empty space, blood and secretions increased, and in the short space of five weeks the patient was cured.

Frederick used at first to vomit much acid matter; later on he vomited whatever he ate or drank. All means were unavailing, and the doctor defined the complaint as induration and contraction of the stomach. This patient's appearance was not sickly, in spite of the features being somewhat aged and the complexion sallow. Much air was expelled from the stomach, he said; the lower body was sometimes distended like a drum, and a pain in the head was of regular occurrence. Here again we have want of activity in the lower regions, indolence of the bowels. Hence the irregular stools, and the accumulation of gases, which occasion the pressure on head and stomach. The patient was made to apply daily, for ten days, a cloth dipped in vinegar-and-water on the abdomen for two hours; daily a warm foot-bath with salt and ashes, and twice every night to wash over his back with cold water. After six days the condition had much improved. After ten days the patient employed twice weekly the short swathing, once the Spanish mantle, and every second day a foot-bath with salt and ashes. The third prescription for the last two weeks consisted in three upper and lower affusions, and two semi-baths reaching to the pit of the stomach. In six weeks the patient was completely restored.

I could quote innumerable such cases: the foregoing may, however, suffice.

Stomach Cramps.

Mr N—— has often had pains in the body from having caught cold. Accumulation of gases in the stomach have caused him to vomit frequently. When much air had been expelled, and he had been able to vomit freely, then he felt relieved, and had an excellent appetite. The complaint, however, went on increasing, and began to return shortly after every meal, with such violence that he sometimes was forced to cry out aloud for pain. His feet and hands were cold, and the body shivering.

In such cases the stomach is mostly quite innocent, pains and vomiting being caused by the violent pressure of the air upon it. Vomiting merely relieves the complaint for the moment, and a complete cure can only be effected by restoring normal and equal heat, and perspiration of the body, and by regulating the circulation.

This was accomplished by washing over the patient

completely with hot water-and-vinegar, three times on the first day as he lay in bed, and, without drying, covering him up to exclude the air. On the second day the process was repeated only twice, and on the third day once. This proceeding suffices whenever a person who has caught cold gets fever combined with vomiting, and with much air expelled from the mouth.

Stomach Tumours.

Violent vomiting, burning pain in the stomach, &c., are yet no positive proof of the existence of stomach tumours, although these are of frequent occurrence.

Such patients should avoid whatever is sour, acid, corrosive, or peppered. Simple diet, and still more simple beverage, have always proved to be the best remedies against incipient tumours. Milk is specially to be recommended.

The treatment of external boils and tumours teaches us to do in like manner with those in the inside. An ulcerated finger may be cured by applying to it a linen rag dipped in cold water, and frequently renewed; and why should not cold water, imbibed half-hourly in spoonfuls, render the same service internally? Instead of water, tea of sage or wormwood may be used, or both together mixed in equal proportions.

A pinch of aloe powder, dissolved in half a pint of water, may be taken in the same fashion, half-hourly in spoonfuls; but never longer than for half a day at a time, with a pause of two or three days before recommencing.

An excellent household remedy, accessible to the poorest, is cabbage-water—viz., the liquid in which cabbage has been pickled. This water will heal the oldest complaints. For this purpose mix one table-spoonful of cabbage-water with six to eight spoonfuls of common drinking-water, and take of it a spoonful every hour.

Ribwort tea is likewise not to be despised. As external applications, I advise such patients to apply a compress on the lower body from one and a half to two hours every second day. A decoction of hay-flowers, shave-grass, or pine-tree will be found still more efficacious than plain water. Large malignant tumours, when once fully developed in the stomach, are incurable. The work of destruction continues to advance, and must infallibly end in death.

Throat Complaints.

Andrew began to relate as follows: "I can hardly speak any more. I had a sore finger. This finger gave me pain the first time I lost my voice; now it begins again to do so. My appetite is good, and nothing is the matter with me. The doctor said the uvula is too long, and must be cut; but I will not consent to this."

The appearance of this man was bloated and inflated, especially the left side of the face from the ear downwards showed a little swelling. It was easy to see that his face was altered, head and neck being inflated both outward and inwardly: this caused pressure, and contracted the inner organs, hence the throat-pains. Evidently the sore finger had not been radically cured the first time—the poisonous matter not entirely removed. To expel this unhealthy matter and cleanse the body is therefore our object; whoever succeeds in doing this will have cured the throat complaint. It will first be necessary to act upon the whole body, and then only to attack the head. To compass the first object, the sack and the shawl are to be employed. Every countryman has a sack at hand. He dips it in a decoction of oat-straw, and puts it on up to the neck. This should be done for three successive days, each time for one and a half hour. After the fourth day let him make use of the sack only every third day; let him wear the shawl daily for one hour. After fourteen days he may begin to employ complete lavations twice in the week, and once weekly a Spanish mantle. If the uvula be still troublesome, let him take a few head vapour-baths, of course on different days. The complaint was entirely removed.

A priest related: "In the course of the summer, 1887, I used to feel an occasional trifling pain in the throat combined with a slight cough. After prolonged preaching, or sitting in the confessional, my voice became gradually weaker and threatened to give way. The complaint increased in September and October. I got a violent catarrh of the throat, and the doctor considered the point of the right lung to be affected. A three months' residence in Meran, gargling and painting the throat, mountain-climbing, &c., all failed to cure me. At last, my leave of absence being nearly up, on the 25th of January I left Meran very despondingly, and repaired to Wörishofen. The cold-water applications—twice daily upper affusion and walking in water — soon brought relief; the pain decreased, the voice became stronger and recovered its former tone, and by Candlemas I was able to hold the service at D———, and deliver a short address from the altar. From week to week I felt improvement. In three weeks' time my voice was as clear and strong as formerly, and I was able to resume all the duties of my vocation."

TYPHUS.

As in smallpox an eruption forms on the surface of the skin, so in typhus we have an internal eruption. According to the seat of this eruption, the malady is designated as typhus of the head or abdomen. In some cases of typhus, outward tumours are also apt to form, but these rarely attain development.

There are three principal points to be observed in the treatment of typhus: firstly, that the fever-heat should never be allowed to reach too high a pitch; secondly, to prevent tumours from forming, and dissolve those already formed; thirdly, as rapidly as possible to remove this poisonous matter from the body.

This threefold object is best attained by means of water, which cools, dissolves, and expels.

John went to the funeral of his brother, who had died of typhus. He imprudently wore a coat which had belonged to the deceased, and within a few days he too was stricken down by the same malady. The heat was great, and greater still the sensation of anxiety and oppression. John ordered a tub of water to be placed near his bed, and whenever the heat and oppression grew unbearable, he entered the tub for one minute. The water reached to the pit of the stomach, and with a coarse towel he rapidly washed over the upper body, then, without drying, he put on a clean shirt and returned to bed. Each time he felt like born anew. He continued to do this for three days, from three to six times in the course of the day. For this he required no clock, but regulated the intervals of his plunges according to the degree of fever-heat. On the first day he bathed six times, on the second three, and the last day only once. In five days all danger was past. But now the convalescent's wife was also attacked by typhus. She too had recourse to the water-tub, and was likewise cured in a few days.

The beverage of both patients consisted of water and curdled milk. They ate nothing until a natural appetite returned, when they partook of bread, soup, milk-soup, and a few potatoes. They were soon able to resume their habitual diet.

During a typhus epidemic, in which within five weeks about twenty persons were treated and saved by means of the aforementioned applications, a little child aged two was also attacked by the malady. No one believed that this fragile creature would be able to survive. Whenever it cried or moaned, the mother dipped it in lukewarm water, with subsequent rapid lavation, or she wrapped the little one in a linen sheet dipped in lukewarm water. In twelve days the child was completely cured.

The coldest water is always the most efficacious; but I sometimes permit the use of lukewarm water for such patients as are likely to be dissuaded from the cure by fear of the unwonted cold shock.

Great panic is generally caused in a school or other such establishment when one of the pupils is attacked with typhus. Without exaggeration, I venture to affirm that if, for instance, of ten children sleeping in one dormitory, one be attacked by typhus, and treated as above, no second child will take the infection. Contagion is mostly conveyed by unhealthy exhalations of the body. According to our method, however, these are absorbed by the wet cloths, and the germs of contagion are thus smothered in the bud. If the apartment is constantly supplied with fresh air, there is little danger of infection being conveyed by the patient's breath. It is hardly necessary, however, to observe that the evacuations of typhus patients should be instantly removed, and, if possible, emptied out at some remote spot.

Ulcers.

A poor labourer had for many months an open sore on the foot, a finger long and three fingers broad. This man, who was in the prime of life, had great and almost continual pain, and could seldom sleep for more than a few hours. His appearance was very sickly, and his courage exhausted. I advised the patient to apply to the sore a plaster made of boiled fenugreek spread upon linen rags; over this to envelop the whole foot above the ankle with fresh coltsfoot-leaves, and then to replace the stocking over everything.

Every morning and evening plaster and leaves were to be renewed; and every two hours he was to swallow two spoonfuls of fenugreek tea. At the same time he was free to pursue his daily occupation. At the end of a fortnight two-thirds of the wound was already healed. The man looked fresh and healthy, and felt no more pain. Three weeks later the foot was completely healed.

The tea of fenugreek is prepared by boiling a small

spoonful of the powdered seeds in a *schoppen* (half a pint) of water for one minute, and then straining.

An official had long suffered from an open sore on the lower part of the calf of the leg. It ulcerated profusely, and the neighbourhood of the spot had assumed a bluish-black hue. This man, whose age might have been about forty-five, was strongly built and rather stout. From his somewhat flushed complexion I recognised him to be a beer-drinker. The eyes were dull, the whites yellowish, the ears dark red. To my question as to his general health he made answer, "There is nothing the matter with me: my appetite is excellent; I am not a drinker, but I enjoy two or three glasses of beer daily. My complaint is a purely local one."

All these patients invariably complain of the one painful or ulcerated spot, believing the cure simply to consist in healing the wound, whereas the treatment should be just the reverse. To heal the body and remove from it all unhealthy matter should be the physician's first task; this once accomplished, the open wound, which is like the entrance to a sewer, will close of its own accord.

If we act otherwise, we thwart Nature, and, so to say, bind her hand and foot, by closing up the sole egress by which the disease could have escaped.

I advised this official for fourteen days to take daily a lower swathing for one and a half hour, and twice daily a complete lavation; in addition to this, every week a head vapour-bath for twenty minutes. These applications had the object of cleansing the body and expelling unhealthy secretions. At the end of fourteen days the official came again to see me. His general health was much improved. The further treatment consisted in two lower swathings weekly for half an hour, and daily one vigorous upper affusion.

On the sore leg nothing was applied but a simple linen rag dipped in lukewarm water, and renewed two or three times daily. After the second fortnight the patient came again rejoicing, for he had now a healthy leg on the healthy body. Since that time he has never ceased to sing the praises of cold water. Those who have thus been cured (and this is important) should continue to practise cold-water applications for some length of time, in order to hinder any new accumulation of unhealthy matter. Let them select those applications from which they have derived most benefit.

As a warning, I will relate the following case: A tolerably stout but very healthy gentleman was afflicted with an open sore on the leg, which gave him much trouble. He had recourse to cold water, and made use of it for twelve days. He could not sufficiently praise its effects; how free and well he felt! If only you would get the troublesome open wound on the leg to close! "Whoever does this will shorten your life," I answered, decidedly. This displeased the gentleman, and he left me. This was in autumn: in the following spring he went, as I heard, to a mineral bath, and after returning home, he employed various means in order to induce the wound to close. He succeeded in doing so, and for six or eight weeks he was able to rejoice in his recovered leg. Then suddenly a large tumour began to form in the middle of the back near the spine. The doctor, believing it to be a boil, attempted to open it by means of a sharp incision, but instead of matter, they came upon a solid hard lump. Within twelve days blood-poisoning had put an end to this vigorous existence.

I might quote many more such instances of similar cases.

Urination, Difficult.

I was once hastily called to a carpenter, seventy years of age, in order to prepare him for death. He had, I was told, fearful pains, and could no longer make water. I soon reached his house; but I could not fulfil my sacerdotal duties, for the man was rushing up and down the room and crying out with pain,—not a minute could he remain quiet. His wife was also crying and lamenting loudly. I directed her to prepare boiling water with a handful of shave-grass, and pour it into the close-stool. It must be remarked that the doctor was two hours off, and would certainly not have found the man alive. The patient seated himself, and allowed the hot vapour to fumigate the painful spots. I ordered him to remain there sitting from twenty to thirty minutes, and then go to bed. In one hour I said I would return and prepare the patient for death. I came at the appointed time, but found the man lying quietly in bed, and in violent perspiration. Joyfully he informed me that two pints of water had gone from him, and he no longer felt the slightest pain. The preparation for death was unnecessary. Next day the man took again a similar vapour application, of twenty minutes' duration; the third day he rested, and on the fourth day resumed his usual work.

The man had caught cold, and thus his complaint had originated. It is incredible what help and relief may be obtained from a simple herb in hours of bitterest suffering.

It may also be recommended, besides the outward application, to drink daily a cupful of shave-grass tea divided in two doses.

A poor labourer suffered from this same complaint, which increased from day to day. He applied shave-grass vapours, but without much effect this time. The vapours alone were too weak, and required to be strengthened by other means. A fourfold linen cloth, dipped in shave-grass decoction, was therefore applied to the affected spot. One vapour application and one such compress daily, applied for two hours, sufficed to cure him in a few days. Catching cold was also here one, though not the sole, reason of the complaint. The water, when voided, showed that much unhealthy matter had been contained in the body.

In a similar case I have employed vinegar-and-water instead of shave-grass with good results.

For all these complaints, as for gravel and stone, an infusion of black-currant leaves is excellent. This tea has often afforded relief even in the severest cases.

Vaccination, Bad Effects of.

A gentleman relates: "I have been healthy all my life. Ten years ago, when smallpox was raging in my neighbourhood, like many others I had myself vaccinated. I got no pustules, but the vaccinated spot on the right arm remained of a reddish colour, and a small eruption came out round the lancet-cuts. For eight years I merely noticed that the inflamed spot continued to grow larger, and now at the end of ten years the moist eruption has become so troublesome that I am sometimes deprived of rest for whole nights. This eruption is stronger now on the one arm, now on the other, and the same change is likewise in the feet. I have tried many remedies, have rubbed the most poisonous ointments on the skin, have taken much medicine, but all in vain."

Here the blood and secretions are certainly corrupted, and the eruption is but an outcome of the unhealthy matter. It is therefore necessary to react upon the whole body, to dissolve and remove whatever is unhealthy in blood and secretions.

Applications—

1. A complete lavation, taken from bed, three times in the week.

2. Washing the eruption two or three times daily with a decoction of fenugreek, or else with a teaspoonful of aloe powder dissolved in a quart of water.

3. Twice weekly a Spanish mantle.

Continue these applications from two to three weeks.

Further applications: Once weekly, or once in the fortnight, a warm bath, with transition into cold. It is also good during this cure to drink tea of wormwood twice daily, each time three or four spoonfuls.

VOICE.

It frequently happens that a person loses his voice, either wholly or partially, without apparent cause.

How can a speaking organ be unfit for use if it be uninjured and free from pain? If I tie a bandage over a person's mouth, he will be unable to speak, and yet his speaking organs are not injured. It would be folly were I to seek the cause of his silence in the throat. I must remove the bandage and speech will be restored.

When idle shepherd boys throw stones into the stream that runs down the valley, and hem its progress with mud and sand, then the water is disturbed from its regular course; it is forced to leave its bed, turning aside to the right or left in order to find a new issue, and sometimes forming stagnant pools in hollows. The same process takes place in the human frame; if we could look into the complicated network of our veins, we should see that just such obstacles are sometimes placed across the passage of our blood, and that agglomerations, swellings of the mucous membranes, &c., are its necessary consequence.

About twelve years ago there came to me a priest who for long had been unable to speak, and had to communicate with his fellow-creatures by means of pencil and paper. Various gargles, caustic, electricity, had all been resorted to without the slightest effect. His general health was good, and he felt no pains; neither was there any perceptible disease to be discovered in the speaking organs. But his complexion wanted freshness, and he had a sickly appearance.

The first upper affusion which I applied revealed to me what mighty agglomerations, almost amounting to tumours, were here existing. These were the culprits which were holding captive the voice with their heavy chains. Remove these, and the voice is free. This result was achieved by means of various applications. The head vapour-bath must first be applied, in order to dissolve the superfluous matter. This produces perspiration over the whole upper body, and the subsequent cold affusion (taken directly after the vapour-bath) carries off that which has been dissolved, and strengthens the whole system. This patient being stout, the determination of blood to the head was averted by means of a vapour foot-bath, succeeded by a cold affusion. These two applications (which in this case were used conjointly) can be taken once in each week; in very stout subjects, as often as twice.

Another application, likewise calculated to dissolve all superfluous matter, is the Spanish mantle; to this are added cold baths (one or two in the week for one minute only), semi-baths reaching to the armpits, with vigorous lavation of the upper body; one upper and one lower affusion may replace the semi-bath.

These applications, punctually performed, and combined with a regular mode of life, plenty exercise, and light manual labour, soon effected the cure, and restored the patient's voice completely, without the assistance of either medicine, burning, or electricity. No one had believed it possible that this priest would regain his power of speech. At the end of six weeks no trace remained of his former complaint; and even now, after a period of twelve years, his voice has a full sonorous tone which rejoices all those that hear it.

A girl, aged sixteen, lost her voice without apparent cause: she was completely hoarse, and could only make herself understood with great difficulty. The doctor had not been able to help her. Her appetite was good, and her appearance blooming: the head somewhat round and full, the short neck slightly inflated. She seemed to breathe with some difficulty. Her feet were always cold.

In six weeks the girl was completely cured. By what means? The blooming complexion, hot and inflated head, and cold feet, showed clearly that she suffered from determination of blood to the head. The principal object to be attained, therefore, was to direct the blood downwards, and restore equal circulation and warmth. The patient took daily two or three cold foot-baths (each one minute in duration), succeeded by exercise in the fresh air. She likewise walked daily on wet stones or in damp grass. These applications were calculated to draw down the blood from above towards the extremities. In order to dissolve and remove the agglomerations in head and throat, the Spanish mantle was used daily during the first week. In the second and third weeks it was only applied every second or third day, and later, only once in the week. After about a fortnight, in order to strengthen the general system, one semi-bath of one minute was taken weekly, in combination with lavation of the upper body. The semi-bath and lavation might likewise have been successfully replaced by an upper and lower affusion.

The restoration of equal warmth was therefore the first, dissolution and removal of unhealthy agglomerations the second, and bracing of the general system the third part of the healing process. The body improved in strength, the voice became clearer and more sonorous than it had ever previously been, and was excellently adapted for singing, an art which the girl continues specially to cultivate.

Worms.

Among the vermin by which our bodies are infected, the ascarides and other sorts of worms are those most calculated to derange and injure the organism. Children are frequently afflicted with them, and if a mother be not careful to notice this, the worms may become very injurious. They are formed in the rectum, and are often caused by eating too much farinaceous food, especially black bread. Worms are usually expelled from below, but may sometimes come out by the mouth. The principal symptoms are: great appetite, uneasiness and pain in the abdomen. When children put their fingers in the nose, it likewise often denotes the presence of worms. The children also look sickly, because the worms rob nature of her proper nourishment.

Remedies against worms are:—

1. Cut up an onion, and place it overnight in a quart of water. In the morning well press out the onion juice, and drink this water fasting. If this remedy be used three or four days in succession, the worms will certainly be killed and expelled.

2. Boil a spoonful of honey in a quart of water and drink it. The worms suck themselves full of this water, and if subsequently a cup of wormwood tea (which is poison to them) be drunk, they will die and come out.

3. The wormseed is the strongest remedy of all for this purpose. It is the seed of a plant thus named, because of its wonderful properties.

Three large worms came one day out of a woman's mouth. She had been ailing for some time, and was taking medicine. Two spoonfuls of wormseed, taken on two consecutive days, had the result of expelling no less than seventy-eight large worms within three days.

Wormseed is not dear, and can be bought in any druggist's.

Of all worms the tape-worm is the most pernicious. Reliable medicines for expelling this reptile can now be obtained in every apothecary's shop, along with the directions for use. Pumpkin-seeds have, however, been known to have the effect of killing and expelling the tape-worm.

INDEX.